IS THAT I

- The title of this book is a reference to some words which Shaun often spoke – mostly when he was delirious – during the final days of his life.

- Any profits consequent upon the sale of this book will be donated to David Cunningham's Research Fund at the Royal Marsden Hospital, Sutton, Surrey.

IS THAT IT NOW?

Sheila Ellesmere

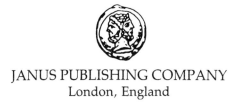

JANUS PUBLISHING COMPANY
London, England

First published in Great Britain 1993
by Janus Publishing Company

Copyright © Sheila Ellesmere 1993

British Library Cataloguing-in-Publication Data.
A catalogue record for this book is available from the British
Library.

ISBN 1 85756 062 0

Cover design David Murphy

Printed & bound in England by
Antony Rowe Ltd, Chippenham, Wiltshire

Contents

Introduction

This book is about grief. The grief that comes to a family when a much-loved member is dying. The grief that comes to a wife and mother as she lives through the months which precede and succeed her husband's death.

Those struggling with grief, or wishing to know how to cope with it, will find comfort and instruction here. But the book is in no way a manual for people wishing to know how to deal with such sadness in their own lives, or anticipating bereavement. It is quite simply one person's unedited reactions and response to the desperate day-to-day events which changed her life. As such, it is what historians call reliable information. It has not been written with any group of readers in mind, nor with the idea of putting forward any particular point of view. Nor does it seek to promote one way of life in preference to another.

But readers will discern that in writing this book the author has had a strong sense of purpose. She gives insights into the sorts of things that happen to a family in these circumstances; the sorts of things which become important and the things which (all of a sudden) are unimportant. How you react when the latest news is bad or during a crisis. And how you respond to such good news as there is. Here, then, is a picture of one family, and their friends from work, school and church, coping with tragedy; one wife and mother living through the final months of her husband's life – and beyond.

These were the months which the couple had been told they had left. Indeed, some of them were a bonus which initial medical predic-

tions did not foresee. Of course, throughout this period there were
great hopes that a recovery might happen – and great sadnesses
whenever such hopes were dashed. Husband Shaun never gave up
hope that a cure would be found. He was fighting right to the end, and
was keen to try any experimental medicine, whatever the discomfort,
which might give him – and those who came next – a better chance.
But the course of his illness – secondary cancer of the liver – was
not, perhaps, radically different from what he and Sheila must have
expected.

This book has the freshness and sharp cutting edge which is so
characteristic of thoughts and experiences which have been put on
paper almost as they happen. In giving these insights, the author
has fashioned a book which becomes, in some way, a celebration of
Shaun's life. The manner in which he coped with his illness; the way
in which he died (which spoke of God's presence); and the reactions
of his friends and family; all demonstrated the sort of man he was.

The book gives well-deserved recognition, too, to the medical prac-
titioners who helped and treated Shaun. It comes through clearly that
the doctors are as thrilled as the people they're seeking to help when
they're able to give good news or renewed hope; and scarcely less sad
than their patients when the news they have to give is bad.

Lastly, of course, this book is about loneliness – the loneliness that
hits you after bereavement. Also the anger – the questions: Why me?
Why us? Why did God choose us for this? And the sadness; the agony
of the first few months. Perhaps readers who have undergone, or are
undergoing, similar experiences will receive some comfort from the
thought – more fully expressed in the author's postscript chapter –
that while the sadness does not go away, and what is past remains
immeasurably precious, it can give way, it does give way, to what is
to come.

1

Shell Shock

How do I start this story? The summer of 1990 – and gall-stones. I was hanging out the washing one July evening when Shaun came home from the doctors' surgery and said that Dr Teed, his soon-to-be-retired GP, thought it was gall-bladder trouble and had given him tablets. I suppose I felt smug. I had said it was probably gall-stones after looking it up in a book at St Francis' school where I teach. A few weeks later the diagnosis changed – cirrhosis of the liver – no drink. Almost immediately after hearing this news, we were off on holiday to Ireland, stopping en-route in Wales with two sets of friends – Roger and Delyth in Creigiau, and David and Ann in Milford Haven. David, a pharmacist, recommended particular tablets for Shaun's stomach ache. I'm glad we had them with us in Ireland for Shaun was not at all well – he was feeling tired and, apart from his continued stomach aches, he was not eating properly.

When we returned, Shaun went to see Dr Powell-Jackson – a specialist – who ordered a scan at the Alexandra Hospital near Maidstone. As a result of that a biopsy was arranged. However, it was put off. Shaun was told there was a possibility of a tumour. Dr Powell-Jackson phoned me at school because I wanted to know why it had been postponed. He said that they had to be very careful – what they thought was a 'secondary' might be enlarged blood vessels and therefore a biopsy might be dangerous. I asked what he meant by 'secondary' and he just said, 'Well, a tumour'.

Another scan was followed a few days later by the biopsy. I think by now I knew it would be cancer, but I was not completely shattered

– after all, this had been found so early, hadn't it? Shaun drove himself
to the Alexandra for the biopsy early in the morning and a good friend
of mine, Noreen, the school secretary, dropped me off there after
school so that I could pick up the car. Shaun was in good spirits,
talking about the long needles being used, and how each one went
deeper and deeper and yet he didn't feel a thing. I picked him up the
following morning and everything seemed fine. An appointment was
made for 5.20 p.m. on September 24th to see Dr Powell-Jackson at the
Maidstone Hospital. Funny, we both left home certain that when we
got there we would be told that Shaun had cancer but that also, if we
did A, B and C, then it would go away and he would be cured.

Nothing prepared me for the truth. I was in a dream world as we
sat there. 'I am sorry but the biopsy shows secondary cancer of the
liver. It has spread from an unknown site, and – I'm sorry – but there
really is nothing to be done. I advise you to go for quality of life as
treatment can be very painful and really has no chance of success.
However, if you like, I can recommend you see Dr Smith (a specialist
in stomach cancer) at the Royal Marsden Hospital, Sutton, Surrey, for
counselling.'

I couldn't stop the tears. Shaun had a wry smile on his face. We
asked how long he had had cancer. Dr Powell-Jackson's reply was
that it was difficult to say but possibly six months – a hazarded guess.
5.20 p.m.: Time etched in my mind forever. I sobbed my heart out in
Shaun's arms in the car park. No way could I go home straight away.
I couldn't drive in the end. Shaun was much stronger than I was. This
was when he started smoking again. Funny, I even remember the
dinner that night – braised steak had been cooking in the slo-cooker
all day – but I don't think it was very tender when I finally dished it
up.

Phone calls came thick and fast and Kathleen's worried face
appeared at the kitchen window as I was washing up. (Kathleen was
a very good friend and neighbour of long standing who had conquered
breast cancer ten years earlier but was now herself suffering from
cancer of the liver.) The whisky came out and we spent a lot of time in
the kitchen. It almost turned into a party! Shell shock had overtaken
us all.

2

Shaun Opts for Experimental Therapy

Monday 8th October

An early morning drive to the Marsden. Lots of traffic. Very busy. When we were almost there, Shaun was saying that the only thing he would consider would be anything experimental. Looking back, I suppose that was a strange thing for him to say when you remember we were only going there for counselling.

We parked and stood there looking at the outside of the hospital when a car drew up.

'Hello Shaun. What are you doing here?'

I didn't know at the time but Steve T. played rugby for Askeans against Shaun's club, Maidstone; Paddy (Shaun's father) was Steve's godfather and had given Steve's mother away at her wedding. Mary, Steve's wife, had cancer and – small world – she was the young Mum who we had been talking about at school as she was being so brave and strong. Shaun made a negative comment about the appearance of the hospital and Mary went for him. She said they were marvellous people and really helpful – something which we came totally to agree with later on. (She also made good comments about St Francis' School.) What a positive outlook she had.

We went in to see Dr Smith. He examined Shaun, spoke to him, and suddenly said that he thought a consultant physician named Dr Cunningham would be interested to see him. We had a half-an-hour wait while David Cunningham was found, and – within five minutes of David examining Shaun and speaking to him – we were caught up on a whirlwind:

'The first thing is, there is no cure, but there is a 50/50 chance of containment. I am experimenting with a new form of chemotherapy using a Hickman line.* I think with your age, fitness and stoical nature it is for you.'

An appointment was fixed for Shaun to go in on Wednesday for two nights. We drove home in a daze. Everything had happened so fast. Dr Cunningham was like a breath of fresh air. He had given us a chance to fight. And fight we would.

Wednesday 10th October

Shaun was driven to the Marsden by his work-colleague, Roger. Our younger son, Stuart, and I went up straight from school to see Shaun. I couldn't believe that he was practising how to inject himself in the stomach! He who had fainted almost at the sight of a dentist's needle? He was in good spirits. The Hickman line was *in* and he was practising how to change the syringe on the pump. Stuart and I drove home in a positive mood.

I collected Shaun on Friday complete with enough medication to fill a whole shelf of the fridge. However, when we got home we were sitting in the garden talking to Frances, a neighbour, when we realised that the pump wasn't working. Frantic phone calls and back to the Marsden on the Saturday morning to collect a new pump. Driving home, we realised that Shaun had not had his tablet, so he made me pull on to the hard shoulder of the M25 motorway as the medicines were in the boot. A police patrol car pulled up behind us; I could see it in my driving mirror but Shaun – bent over the boot of the car looking for the right tablet to take – was completely oblivious until the policeman put his arm on his shoulder and asked *me* if I was alright. Shaun said to him, 'It's alright, I'm just looking for my drugs!' The officers were very polite; they obviously believed us, although we had many a chuckle about it afterwards.

---

* This is a form of chemotherapy in which a tube is inserted into the main vein in the chest. This is connected to a syringe which the patient carries, normally in a pouch or a 'bum bag' around his waist. The syringe contains a special mixture of chemotherapy operated by a syringe driver – a form of battery-operated pump. The whole thing works on a timer so that a controlled dose of chemotherapy is administered constantly. Syringes, of which we kept a regular supply in the fridge, had to be changed every 24 hours.

There followed a pattern. Every third week Shaun went to Out-patients to see David Cunningham, and every fourth week for an overnight stay for a 'platignum wash through' (the platignum being fed into his system through a drip feed). He always felt very well over the weekend following these treatments. I would leave school Friday lunchtime and drive to the Marsden to collect him. If we hurried the pharmacist, we could just make the Angel at Addington for a quick drink before they closed. Often we met friends, Don and Margaret C., and then we would collect Stuart from school. Nice times, happy memories.

3

New Routines sometimes have Hiccups

Over the weeks we got used to administering the treatment. Shaun used to dread Mondays, Wednesdays and Fridays, as these were the nights on which he had to take the drug, Interferon. We would set everything up on the dining room table and he would have to carefully mix the drug with the special water. He was really very brave about it and at first he did very well. It was only later on that he sometimes had problems. He knew that he must not inject into the bloodstream and I think this played on his mind so much that he became frightened. On those nights we rang the twilight (ready-call) nurses and they were marvellous. They never ever got to do his injections because it seemed that once they were in the house all Shaun's confidence returned and he injected himself with ease. Another problem with the Interferon was its side effects. It could give flu-like symptoms so Shaun took paracetamol on those nights. These symptoms meant he had to start taking time off work to recover. (Shaun's work normally took him to the head office of Leadenhall Motor Policies at Lloyds where he worked as a Motor Insurance Underwriter.)

Changing the pump became a chore as well, not so much for Shaun but more for me. Not that I ever did it – he always did it himself – but I spent my time worrying that the battery would run out, or that the syringe wouldn't last through to the next change, or even that it wouldn't stay attached properly. We did have a couple of scares. The first was while we were spending a long weekend in Stratford-on-Avon for our 24th wedding anniversary. Shaun had changed the pump when we returned from the cinema after watching *Memphis*

Belle. However, after I had been asleep for several hours I woke up to
find Shaun looking at his Hickman line, the tube of which was full of
blood. He had forgotten to clamp it off after changing the pump earlier
on and therefore, instead of the treatment being forced up the tube, it
was releasing blood downwards. Shaun was not a bit bothered. 'It
doesn't matter,' he said. I was the one who panicked. He cleaned the
line out and calmly went back to sleep, leaving me a nervous wreck.
After that I used to drive him crazy every night saying, 'Have you
clamped?' He would get very cross with me!

The other accident he had with the pump was not, thank goodness,
witnessed by me. I had already left for school, leaving Shaun eating
his breakfast and waiting for Roger to pick him up for work. Apparently the pump had become detached and Shaun looked down to find
his shirt covered in blood. He said it looked as though he had been
shot in the stomach! I'm not sure what Roger's feelings were, walking
in on this. Anyway, Shaun changed the line, adding a new clamp,
and put his once-white shirt into the sink to soak. Remember, I still
didn't know anything about this, and Shaun went gaily off to work. It
wasn't until half-way through the morning that he realised that I
would arrive home before him and would probably get the fright of a
lifetime to find the bloodstained shirt. So, he came home from work
at lunchtime to wash the shirt and get rid of the evidence before I
could even get to know about the incident. That was typical of his
caring, thinking attitude towards me. He was right, I would have
imagined the worst!

A pattern set in with the treatment; it became almost second nature,
although I still looked for the little flashing light on the pump continually which would reassure me that everything (at least equipment-
wise) was working properly. At night, when he got up to go to the
loo, it would look like aeroplane landing lights flashing around the
bedroom.

Shaun quite looked forward to the overnight stays. He always felt
so well after the platignum wash throughs and they always resulted
in good weekends. The tiredness which had been dogging him did
not happen after these stays and he was always so bright. He enjoyed
the visits from elder brother Terry and his wife, Geraldine, and old
friend, Hank, and the resultant drinking sessions. They obviously
helped the treatment to be washed through! I asked Hank to give his
impressions of these visits and I shall insert them here:

'The first time I visited Shaun at the Royal Marsden I was filled with some trepidation. I did not really know the extent of his illness or, therefore, the state I would find him in, but, in the end, the occasion passed by as a very pleasant surprise. Although having previously lived in the area for 20 years I was somewhat amazed to discover that the hospital was actually situated where it was, and even then I missed the main entrance on my first approach! Arriving at the hospital later than most visitors, I found the lower corridor was deserted, and the first person I actually saw was on the floor of Shaun's ward.

Shaun took no time to find. He was in the first room on the left. There was only one other occupant of the room but he remained asleep for the next two hours. It was good to see that Shaun, although attached to pumps and drips, was very much the Shaun of old. In fact, armed with a book and a newspaper, he seemed quite content watching the golf on television. There was only one thing missing . . . I quickly remedied the situation by producing an evening's supply of canned bitter. The fact that all Shaun's urine was to be tested did not unduly concern the very pleasant nursing staff who allowed all refreshments to be imbibed without hindrance.

To be honest, Shaun was in good form, although I gather he was always a bit down in the days following the treatment – probably a hangover! The evening passed quickly but frequently interrupted by Shaun's collecting of samples in the very handily adjacent loo. However, by half-way through the visit the 'bedside method' was more favoured, thus removing the risk of tripping over the various tubes in the proximity.

I hope Shaun enjoyed the visit because, for me, the evening had been very good. It would perhaps be nice to record that it had been a riotous occasion, full of laughs, but it was not always quite like that. Company, a chat, a drink and the best of friendship were all that I could offer at a time when I felt particularly helpless.

Subsequent visits were much the same. The room changed; so too did the other occupants. Shaun was very critical of those patients who did not attempt to encourage their visitors. He was also very keen to express his gratitude to all the people around him; obviously family but also to his employers who made his visits to the Royal Marsden so much easier. His trust in the hospital staff also was very obvious.

By the time of my final visit Shaun had gained his single room. (As a BUPA patient he had expected this from the start.) Often his greatest concern was that the treatment should begin and finish in time for him to return to Kent by lunchtime the following day before "last orders" was called. But seriously, I think Shaun did become more frustrated as time went by although certainly, in my company, he always retained a very positive attitude towards the future, for which I will always remain grateful.'

It was during this period that Dr Cunningham added a mild dose of Warfarin to the treatment. This must have had the effect of thinning the blood because Shaun began to feel the cold and I eventually went out to buy him three pairs of pyjamas – something new!

Christmas 1990

We were determined to have a really good Christmas and we did. The house seemed continually full of visitors and we did enjoy ourselves in spite of the underlying worries. We took many photos and Shaun looked good in them all. He was a born fighter, always so positive that he would really fight this thing hanging over us. The pattern continued much as before, alternating between tiredness, feeling well, having to have some time off work. New Year's Day arrived and Stuart broke his leg while playing football, wearing his birthday presents of a goalkeeper's jersey and goalkeeper's gloves. I remember Shaun saying to me, while lying on the settee, 'You'd better take him for an X-ray although he's probably only sprained it.' Shaun thought that casualty would be empty on this of all days but of course it wasn't. They were short-staffed, though, and as I held Stuart's leg while the nurse plastered it, my back went! There was now no way I was fit to go back to school at the beginning of term and I went to our new GP, Dr Gardner, to ask for a week off. He insisted I take a month – I think, probably, more because of my mental state than anything else. I eventually took the time off gratefully, much to Shaun's surprise. It gave me much more peace of mind to be at home with him. Sometimes during this period he was going to work as normal – he was not going to give in. Sometimes he was just too tired to move.

It was now that I thought about keeping a diary and I began to wish I had started it earlier. Originally I had thought that all would be well but now I was not making any long-term plans, although we were receiving so much positive help in the form of a veritable bombardment of Mass Cards and prayers. God must have wanted him so much. These tokens from people were so uplifting to us both; how do people go through life without thinking of God? I know He has sustained us so well. The chapters that follow are largely a transcript of my diary, which Shaun knew I was keeping but which he didn't want to read. He knew I was suffering and there was absolutely nothing he could do about it except continue with his positive attitude. That he surely did; he never ever gave up, not even at the end.

4

January 1991 – Renewed Hopes and Fears

Tuesday 22nd

Are all the stomach aches and pains and tiredness related to the treatment? Or the cancer? Is the Warfarin really necessary? He feels the cold so much. How long have we got? If it's the treatment that's causing all the pain, is it worth us *all* suffering?

What is the treatment doing? Is it just prolonging the inevitable? Therefore is it worth him feeling so bad all the time? Would it be better to opt for quality?

The steroids? Are these the cause of depression and the heightening of all aches and pains?

How can I cope? If he is down or suffering then so am I. What can I do to be strong?

We were told the side effects would be minimal. True or false? I never thought of Shaun as having a low pain threshold. He was forever saying to the boys when they were younger and hurt themselves, 'It's only pain!'

Wednesday 23rd

Shaun actually got up at 11.00 a.m. today. He says he is feeling slightly better than yesterday. Fiona, the ready-call nurse, came for the injection. Her husband has broken his leg! Shaun did his injection with no problem. Still having constant stomach aches.

Thursday 24th

Royal Marsden today for the sixth course of treatment. Jack, the Leadenhall driver, arrived about 9.30 a.m., but Shaun not very well. Worried, I think, about the scan. Rang from the Marsden about 11.15 a.m. – own room being prepared, sounds down. I phoned after 5.00 p.m. and Shaun sounded more cheerful. Has had a sleep and they have started the treatment already.

9.30 p.m.: Shaun has phoned. David Cunningham says scan to be done next week – and that he will stop the treatment as the tumour is static. Not got as small as he had hoped. Can it now hold its own without treatment or has the treatment to be shuffled about to try again later? David Cunningham's reaction to the stomach pains: 'I might as well shut up shop as I am causing everyone pains!'

How does Shaun feel about coming off the treatment? He's not sure. How do I feel? Don't really know – as long as his pains clear up and as long as he is monitored closely!

Friday 25th

Funny how I feel on tenterhooks, waiting for the time to come to drive to the Marsden.

Anyway, Stuart and I left about 11.00 a.m. and there really wasn't any problem. Shaun was standing on his balcony when we arrived. We had about a half-an-hour wait and saw Andrea, a sister, who had burnt her fingers on hot oil while frying prawns in a wok!

Anyway we had plenty of time to make the Angel – first time Stuart had been with us. I think he quite enjoyed the outing as well. Shaun has been quite bright for the rest of the evening. I cancelled the twilight nurse. Nice thought for Shaun – a rest from the injections! I am feeling better as well. Incredible how my morale is so wrapped up with his. Natural really, I suppose.

Tidings of Hope

Saturday 26th

Shaun went back to bed after breakfast and I went shopping. Later on he enjoyed a bath – something he has not been able to do recently.

Then the most incredible thing happened. Monica B. phoned and asked if Shaun and I would like to go to Lourdes at Easter. (Monica had been helping to organise and raise funds for these Easter trips for years.) We were stunned – had never dreamt that it would be possible. Another great morale booster. Shaun first of all felt embarrassed, but we will go! The boys say we should. Feel much more uplifted – some good news in January after all! Nick, my youngest brother, wife Sue and daughter Lizzie arrived about 5.30 p.m. and stayed until 7.00 p.m. They brought beautiful daffodils and an Irish song cassette tape for Shaun.

Sunday 27th

Michèal, priest from St Francis' Church, arrived at 10.00 a.m. just before we went to Mass. I knew he must have recommended Shaun to Monica! He picked up our portable phone and thought he would give himself a laugh. He phoned Tricia (a fellow teacher of mine at St Francis' School) pretending he was on a car phone on the middle of the M25! Shaun took our elder son, Matt, for another driving lesson. He says he is doing well. I phoned Monica – she says she is really pleased we have accepted.

Wednesday 30th

I don't really believe it. Shaun has had two really good days and then – last night – he was really freezing. Stomach pains have started up again. No way could he get up for work today. I rang to tell Roger, and then Lionel, Shaun's boss, rang us from Edinburgh and, later his wife, Elizabeth, rang. My Mum and Dad came; the train was late, so they missed the connection. Got back here about 12.00 noon – Shaun still in bed; he had forgotten they were coming. He got up at about 1 o'clock but spent most of the time on the settee. His stomach, he says, is tender all over, not just the tumour. Why??? I think there are three possible answers although Shaun doesn't agree with me. He is very depressed – talking about getting on a dangerous flight with a view to it being bombed. My opinion: maybe the treatment isn't yet out of his body, maybe it is the actual tumour or maybe it is muscle tension caused by the depression and anger. How such a change can take place so quickly in a person is incredible. It affects us all, though.

Yesterday Shelagh O., a friend and fellow teacher, came to lunch and said how well I looked (and I certainly felt it). Today it's a different story!

5

February – a Break from Treatment but not from Pain

Sunday 3rd

I've felt really down today. Crazy isn't it? Probably because of the messing around over the last few days. On Thursday I took Shaun to the Marsden – 1.00 p.m. He had an appointment for the scan but it was 2.30 p.m. before we went in. I had planned on finding Sister Andrea while he was having it done, to sort out pain killers for Shaun's stomach. I went up to Mayneord Ward and they bleeped her, but there was no answer – so after 20 minutes I went back to Shaun. He was still waiting to be given his stuff to drink so I tried Miles Ward. The sister there said Andrea was shopping but she bleeped the doctor. He wanted to see Shaun after his scan. Anyway, Shaun's scan took 35 minutes – they took 66 pictures – Shaun had counted 82 but he said, 'Never mind, '66 was a good year!' (World Cup win and we got married!). Saw the doctor and he gave us some strong pain killers. Got home to Stuart eventually at 4.45 p.m. Friday morning Stuart had to get up early – appointment at fracture clinic at 9.30 a.m. Eventually seen (for a few minutes)! We are to come back in two weeks. Finally got home at 11.30 a.m.

Saturday: Shaun seemed alright at breakfast but then went back to bed for the morning. He watched the rugby in the afternoon. We went to The Wheelers pub and again he seemed alright – Paula and Jim, the licencees there, are giving up their tenancy in June. The walk home, however, wore Shaun out – he ate his supper and fell asleep. Went to bed early. Today, after a wakeful night, he got up for breakfast and then went back to bed. He didn't come to Mass. I felt alright in church – went slowly downhill after that, probably because Shaun didn't rouse himself until gone 1 o'clock and then he was crabby. He literally stood on the patio for two minutes and then came in. The sum total of his fresh air for the day! He fell asleep after dinner. I went up to bed in a bad mood. Josephine (neighbour Frances' daughter) called in later – I like talking to her. Talked about her sister Marian's cottage near Caen – sounds nice. Shelagh Mc., an old school friend, phoned later – she thinks it's early days for Shaun to have his strength back. She will make some enquiries about this. All I know is that I am fed up. Am I doing the right thing by going back to work tomorrow? My back is twingeing now on the other side and poor Stuart will be bored to tears. How much more can I take?

The big freeze of 1991

Thursday 7th

Only 20 children in school today, due to the snow. Four only left by 1.30 p.m. School was closed and will be tomorrow. I was worried about Shaun and Roger driving to the Marsden due to the conditions, but the motorway was fine – they did get stuck on Chatham Hill for one and a half hours, though, trying to get back to work. Good news, anyway! Dr Cunningham is pleased with the build-up of calcium which he thinks means the cancer cells are dying and Shaun has eight weeks free from treatment. He will have the Hickman line taken out next week so he can then come off the Warfarin. Prayers of thanks now, but also for the future.

Mortar bombs attacked Whitehall today. Matt, who works as a civil servant in Whitehall, said they were evacuated into the street but that no check was made on names or numbers. That is very worrying.

Poor Shaun had to visit the loft complete with hairdryer to defrost the pipes as we had no cold water left in the tank. No wonder he is tired tonight. Carmel, a headmistress and friend from my college days, has phoned – she has staffing problems.

Saturday 9th

Stuart and I watching a video, *Always*. He has never heard of Purgatory – which I think is relevant to the film. However, I am convinced that

Purgatory is here on earth – especially after the months since last September! Shaun went back to bed after breakfast – I went to town through the snow and although he said he was going for a cat-nap he was still asleep when I got back after 12.00 noon! He blames the good breakfast! He began to clear the snow but got too tired. He went to bed about 9.00 p.m. I hope his strength comes back. I empathise with jockey Bob Champion, and hope his story comes true for us – Shaun feels he's dying during the treatment, alright while off it! Mike, my brother, phoned from Perth, Australia, where he lives, to see how Shaun got on on Thursday. Lovely!

Sunday 10th

A good day, with a very good beginning! First try for months! We went (walked) to 9.00 a.m. Mass later. Shaun hasn't had a bad day. He has lasted out well although he went to bed at about 9.45 p.m. No school tomorrow due to wintry weather.

Monday 11th

Another good morning – awake early – and another try. We'll get there! No school again due to snow. Got a taxi cab to Safeway and in the afternoon walked into town. Got Stuart tracksuit/shell suit bottoms for when his plaster comes off. Phoned the Marsden to get Shaun's Hickman line removal appointment – not till next week. Also spoke to Dr Gardner regarding pain killing tablets. Hard work getting past the young receptionist! Matt didn't go to London – British Rail have 60% of their rolling stock out of action on the Southern Region. Wrong Snow! Really bad weather. Bought Shaun a tonic from my friendly pharmacist.

Wednesday 13th

The meeting of Fr Chris (Priest at St Francis' Church) and Lionel went well! An inter-church football match might result from their meeting. Bad school day today. Mr D. (our head teacher) and Noreen on a course – two school buses not in. Only the Bearsted one arrived –

brought in about a dozen children. Ash Wednesday, school to finish
at 2.00 p.m. but parents of children in the Annexe (for infants) were
not informed!

Fr Chris arrived at 5.20 p.m. – Shaun and Lionel not home until an
hour later. Cheese and pickle sandwiches all round. Lionel going to
his church service. Friend and hairdresser, Pauline, came to cut our
hair – Shaun still very tired. Last night he slept from 7–11.00 p.m.,
and then all night!

Friday 15th

Stuart had his plaster off this morning and the X-ray seems okay. He
is now wearing a tubi-flex and can only put a little weight on his foot
while indoors. Had to get minicabs there and back due to ice on the
road. Jack took Shaun to the Marsden to have the Hickman line
removed. He had to wait until nearly lunch time before Dr Finlay was
able to do it. The local anaesthetic, he was told, would feel like bee
stings, and Shaun said one did hurt. The doctor had quite a job to get
the Hickman line out. Shaun reckons he could feel himself being
pulled up as the doctor tugged and tugged. Afterwards, Dr Finlay
was sweating and said it was the toughest one he had ever had to do!
Funnily enough they haven't stitched the hole where it went into his
chest and it is leaking slightly.

I feel down and depressed again tonight – don't like the thought of
blood. I'm worried about both Stuart and Shaun. I've got to get out of
these *down* moods.

Saturday 16th

Funny – or hard – the feelings you get. If Shaun has to die before the
allotted three score years and ten is it right to try to 'buy' the extra few
years now? At least I could maybe pick up the pieces and make
something, albeit for myself, for the rest of my life? I wish I knew
exactly *how* long we have. Alright, last September 24th I didn't even
dare envisage Christmas 1990, but now we're talking about the wedding of Veronica (daughter of friends of ours) in September 1991. *But*
– and it's a *big but* – I don't want to see him suffer. I think he has had –
and is going through – a lot of pain. What on earth will it be like before
he finally dies? There, I've finally said it – 'die'. How will I cope?

Rather now than later? I don't know, really. Friends Dave and Mary arrived after delivering their daughter Claire to Gatwick. Really cheered me up after this morning's unsatisfactory School Governors' meeting. Broke down with Mary this evening – she says I need my own space. Shaun enjoyed it while they were here although he was tired by about 10.00 p.m.

Tuesday 19th

Haven't felt like writing for a few days. Shaun was really bad on Sunday – so depressed. Had his breakfast and then stayed in bed until after 1.00 p.m. Bad mood all day, culminating in the evening when I asked how he was, with the reply, 'No, I'm not alright. I've got cancer!' Monday morning he was talking about six months' sick leave followed by packing up work altogether. I felt down. He came home a lot more cheerful, saying he had perked up at lunchtime. I can't switch moods so quickly. Still feel miserable – and hard-done-by! How selfish of me!

A new motor for the washing machine will cost £95.

Shaun is worried tonight about the number of pain killers he needs. I privately agree – next step morphine? And then what? *I don't want him in pain!!*

Thursday 21st

Big article in the *Daily Mail* about a man who died five years ago. He had exactly what Shaun has. Shaun read it and smiled ironically; good breakfast time reading, he said! He certainly has been happier over the last few days. I wish I could cheer up – I feel trapped with poor old Stuart still stuck here, although I did actually go to Mass and then had lunch with our good friend Rose in The Badger and Honeypot in Maidstone. Trouble is, I felt guilty leaving Stuart! Matt has been quiet for a few days – I think the travelling is getting him down. Cancellations last week because of snow, then the bomb at Victoria on Monday and the hoax phone calls since. Went to see neighbour Kathleen's daughter, Teresa, after her appendix operation and they say Kathleen is very confused. It doesn't sound good. Met Sister Mary in town – says she is glad we are going to Lourdes. Altogether 12 of us are going.

Friday 22nd

Started off very well with verbal promises of a good weekend to come! Took Stuart to fracture clinic. More exercises can be done now and he can start to put weight on it. Spoke to Shaun on the phone this afternoon and worried slightly as he said he had had a few pints at lunchtime as Eddie was down from the Edinburgh branch of Shaun's company. He felt fine. I wondered about the effect on him for the weekend – especially after the few drinks last Saturday. Anyway, he walked home from The Running Horse, early. Lionel would be cross if he knew because he had told Shaun to phone me for a lift. I took him down to Dr Gardner to get a letter of eligibility for Lourdes and to have his stitches out. No waiting necessary – Dr Gardner said he looked remarkably well. Later in the evening, however, the stomach pains were back. Is it the bitter? I have a sinking heart.

Saturday 23rd

I suppose we're all on short fuses! What you think will be a nice evening can turn sour. Take-away meal, a bottle of wine and a video was the setting, but the video (*War of the Roses*) wasn't any use and Shaun was short tempered while the boys (Stuart and his friend) made noises eating prawn crackers. Because the boys were downstairs Shaun made it obvious that he needed to be alone before he went upstairs. I rowed with him – the niceties of life have still to be observed – but Stuart wondered what he had done wrong.

Far cry from this morning when success after five months was achieved. Not great elation however on his side.

Things have started to dawn on Stuart. He asked me for – and gave me – a cuddle. I think he might now realise how serious things are.

Monday 25th

I don't really know what to write. Yesterday started off alright. Shaun and I went to 9.00 a.m. Mass and Fr Jim (St Francis' Parish priest) spoke very emotionally about the war in the Gulf. Shaun then took Matt for a driving lesson and they bought roofing felt for the shed. They spent an hour or so fixing it but then he went slowly downhill getting very crabby after dinner. I shouted at him, saying he was on a

short fuse. I shouldn't have done it, but there are four of us to consider.
I have hated the last two weekends. Miserable.

Shaun had a bad night – even a nightmare which he remembers
nothing about. He was depressed this morning – couldn't go to work,
feels that the swelling is growing. Says that sometimes he feels he has
a brick in his stomach, other times a pebble. I think more and more
about Beachy Head – good job I'm *only* thinking, I suppose!

Tuesday 26th

Shaun still depressed and with pains in his stomach again. Didn't go
to work.

Kathleen died at 1.15 p.m. today. Teresa came up tonight to tell me.
Although I was expecting it, I am still so upset. She was like a beacon
for us – so good, yet really human. Her saying for anyone who had
not pulled their weight: 'Bad luck on him, I say!' Pneumonia was the
final straw for her. Can't help personalising her death, her situation –
it's far too close to home. Funny, I know she's laughing at me now,
telling me probably to have a whisky! I hope, really hope – *but I really
know and trust* – that she has her reward, and everything has got to be
so much better than in her wildest dreams. Peace, greatest peace for
her; hurt and torment for those left behind.

A question on the night of Kathleen's death: Is it worth the treatment
and the suffering involved for the patient when *it* is going to get you
in the end? Who are we kidding? Should we just go with God's will,
not inflict treatment? Who are we prolonging it for? We (as a family)
suffer during the prolonging as well, even though we have the hope
of an outright cure. Again, who are we kidding? Only ourselves.

We *know* when they are dead they are better off, but what they have
given us on this earth, in this life, is what we miss – cannot do without
– and it's *this* that makes us selfish and collapse or indulge in grief.

6

March – a Bad Start to a Good Month

Friday 1st

Shaun has had the whole week off work. The Marsden told him to see
Dr Gardner to find a stronger pain killer. He has told Shaun to *up* the
dose of co-proximal – and if that doesn't work he has given him DHC
(dihydrocodeine). He says his stomach is really tender – gone to bed
early again.

10.15 p.m.: Shelagh Mc. has phoned. She recommends trying the new
tablets, but if they get rid of the pain and really knock him out, then
an in-between strength tablet is available. It is a question, I suppose,
of trial and error. I feel miserable and am dreading another weekend
like the last two. Stuart was back to the fracture clinic today. Physio-
therapy is now to be arranged and I think we will try school on
Monday. I can't help asking myself: if Shaun is suffering now – and
me too! (there I go being selfish again) – how much worse will it get,
and will I be able to cope?

Met Monica at the hospital. She talked about the people going to
Lourdes.

I wish I could express my true feelings.

Now slightly worried about Matt. He's not in and it's 11.00 p.m. He
rang Shaun and said he would be late – someone's birthday – but I
thought I would see him before this.

Monday 4th

Beginning to wonder whether I ought to stop this diary – it's full of moans and misery. Shaun hasn't improved with the new tablets – even when he takes paracetamol as well. Going back to Dr Gardner tomorrow. It is getting me down. Caught myself thinking about the future at one point today – and the picture was of a very lonely Christmas. I don't think I can take it sometimes. I shall miss the companionship and camaraderie – and the odd argument! It's just the thought of Shaun not being there any more. My friend.

Wednesday 6th

Shaun has been really bad today. Sharp pain which started in the kidney area and pain when passing water. Dr Johnson, a partner in our local GP's practice, has taken a sample but we can't wait for that. Kathleen's funeral was beautiful. Uplifting in a funny way. But Shaun couldn't stand up for much of it. I brought him home but he couldn't lie in bed; I had him propped up. Rang David Cunningham's secretary and I am taking him in tomorrow. I hope they can help him – I hate seeing him in pain – and this is the worst I think he's been. I don't know about Lourdes even – whether we will make it.

Took Stuart for his first physio and he actually got his knee to a 90 degree angle.

Doctor Cunningham to the Rescue

Sunday 10th

I'll try a resumé of the past few days as the change round is quite spectacular. Dr Cunningham has got to be brilliant. Within a few minutes of listening to Shaun's symptoms, he knew exactly what was wrong: capsulitis – inflammation of the area surrounding the liver. He gave Shaun antibiotics, steroids and anti-fungal tablets and said they would work quite quickly. Shaun was a lot better by Friday evening – Ann D., a former work colleague of his, was here when I got home. Saturday morning and Florrie (Shaun's Mum) was on the phone again, very upset. Mother's Day this weekend and Florrie's close friend, Kathleen, would be at her daughter's. We arranged to meet her at the cemetery, only she forgot! Found her in her local club, the Newbridge. Saw Mum and Dad and it pleased them to see Shaun.

Shaun and I went to The Wheelers in the evening and had a very enjoyable evening and night.

The steroids have caused a great turn round!

This morning we went to 9.00 a.m. children's Mass and posies were given to the Mums. Five girls from my class brought me posies. Quite a tear-jerker!

Matt went off to watch Spurs play – at least they won.

Shaun and I went to the presbytery tonight for a discussion about the Lourdes pilgrimage. Everything seems in hand.

Going back to last Thursday, while we were waiting to see David Cunningham, an older man, obviously a surgeon, went rushing into David's room – 'Bloody marvellous', he said, and they both congratulated each other. D. C. said they were really pleased – a woman had been referred to them from another hospital with an enormous stomach tumour, having been told that nothing could be done for her.

David Cunningham said they work as a team – David shrank the tumour right down with chemotherapy and the surgeon then cut it out. If only liver cancer could be dealt with in the same way!

Matt seems very down and extra quiet at the moment – it worries me.

Take Stuart for physio at 8.00 a.m. tomorrow!

Thursday 14th

Gaps in the diary – a sure sign that things are going so well. I think Shaun is stronger now than he has been since before we went to Ireland. He has done a lot of gardening and is building up his stamina day by day. Shaun's former work colleague, Tony S., came to see him on Monday and Mìchèal did some muck spreading in the garden yesterday.

Jack took Shaun to the Marsden today and they were pleased with him. Has 10 days of reducing steroids to take and then we'll see if he can cope on his own.

Saturday 16th

There is a man sitting opposite me at the table tonight; he has just eaten a Chinese take-away meal and is talking on the phone to work colleague Palo – and there is *no way he is dying from cancer!* Thank God!

Have just braved a thunder storm to get to The Wheelers early because Matt is attending a wedding evening and he has to get a train.

Shaun has been so good this week. I hope God is listening when I say a great big *Thank You!*

Sleeplessness

Thursday 21st

Shaun worked half days Monday, Tuesday and Wednesday this week but didn't go in today. This not being able to sleep at night is becoming wearing. He gets up and comes downstairs for an hour or so. His mind is buzzing. What to do in the garden? All the names of the various plants? What improvements to make in the house? He reminds me of what they say about a woman a week before she gives birth – over-active, doing everything. I hope that subconsciously he is not trying to cram everything possible into a short space of time . . .

He has the beginnings of a stomach ache again tonight. I worry. I don't want him in pain.

Friday 22nd

Had to smile when we woke up. Shaun said he was pleased with himself because he had had four hours' sleep!

He wandered around town in the morning, had coffee in Waterstone's in Maidstone and met me for lunch. We had French onion soup and a roll in The Badger and Honeypot and then he went to buy pansies for the tree stump in the garden. It looks good. I could get used to these lunch hours. He has gone to The Wheelers for a couple with Pauline's husband, Ron – but he has been out for more than three hours!

Sunday 24th

A different weekend. When Matt came home on Friday night it was to announce that he and Jo are together. We are pleased – we've seen it coming longer than they have! On Saturday Josephine and Max called in with photos of the French cottage. Looks nice. I then drove Jo up to Penenden Heath and let her talk. She was worried about telling Ann and David but I kept telling her I knew they would understand.

We went to Raffles and had a smashing time with Shelagh and Pete Mc., and Matt and Jo took a cab to The Bull at Linton.

This morning the boys came to the 9.00 a.m. Palm Sunday Mass with me and then we picked up Jo. Eventually she spoke to Ann and David and they are thrilled to bits; they also had seen it coming. Jo must feel better now.

Tuesday 26th

Shaun drove himself to the Marsden today – his stomach is starting to hurt and is swollen. David Cunningham thinks the capsulitis is not completely cleared up. Shaun had a big shot of chemotherapy which is making him sweat a lot. He also has more steroids to take.

Jo is not staying tonight. She is going to a family friend. Lionel called in on his way back to Bristol with lots of work for Shaun. He mustn't overdo it. Lionel will take us to (and collect us from) Gatwick.

Wednesday 27th

What a good night!

Friday 29th

Shaun has been much better. He met me for lunch yesterday and we met friends Bob and Linda.

Matt and Jo phoned from Wales last night – they sound happy. Today I was upset when I read the papers and saw that Ralph Bates, the former actor and well-known personality, had died of pancreatic cancer.

This afternoon Shaun and I ordered a three-piece suite. Cost a fortune!

Sunday 31st

Went to Nick and Sue's today. Mum and Dad as well. Very enjoyable.

We have packed and are ready to take off for Lourdes in the morning.

Took Stuart to Alice's tonight.

Phyllis, a friend whose son died tragically in 1990, was so upset in Mass this morning. Said she felt very sorry for me. I feel for her.

Lots of phone calls including one from my mother-in-law (Mum E.); upset because Shaun's brother Terry is off to Devon; also Carmel, Joy and Rose.

7

April – Lourdes and Beyond

Tuesday 9th

Nine days since my last diary entry. But we had a marvellous time in Lourdes. Shaun was so well. He was pushing wheelchairs up the mountain-side, not sitting in them himself. We were both so impressed with the hard work and caring attitude of the helpers. The whole atmosphere of the place is wonderful. Coming back on the plane Shaun said it was the best holiday we've had.

Shaun is now working mornings only. His only problem at the moment is the steroid reaction – the puffy cheeks and swollen stomach which he finds uncomfortable. His appointment with David Cunningham has been postponed until the 18th April. I dread the thought of him going back on the Hickman line treatment. He is more philosophical.

Have been decorating the living room – feel tired – could be the change of air from last week.

Wednesday 10th

11.30 p.m.: I can't believe I'm going to lose him! I **need** him here with me! Being without Shaun is not worth thinking about. I couldn't possibly be me if he wasn't here. I need him in order to function. I want to go first – but I must see the boys settled happily first so that they only have happy memories. I can't be doing with them being upset as well.

(Joked with Shaun tonight about listening to babies' heart beats or feeling them kick – because of the size of his stomach.) Thinking that at the moment things are similar to being pregnant – his waking up so often at night; me, being a mother and a light sleeper, wake up every time Shaun stirs. (At least Shaun has steroids to back him!)

Sunday 14th

Shaun is really uncomfortable with his stomach. It is getting him down and making him irritable. There is also a funny tent-shaped lump in the middle of his stomach. Worrying, when you don't know what it is.

I dread the thought of him resuming treatment. If only the laser could be properly working and guaranteed to kill off the wretched tumour.

I must try and stay positive. It would be marvellous if we could keep the Lourdes feeling for ever.

Finished decorating the lounge yesterday. Jo moved to her bedsit and came here to dinner.

Spurs won the semi-final at Wembley.

Went to 6 p.m. Mass tonight (where I gave the reading). Spoke to Phyllis and her husband Henry. I did think a lot about them while in Lourdes.

Thursday 18th

Shaun went to the Marsden today. I had worried all day about him going back on the Hickman line and all the problems (particularly the injections) this would involve. But the news was different. David Cunningham says the treatment has stopped working and he is now going to try a weekly drip of carbo-platin. The tent-shaped lump is a hernia caused by the steroids. Shaun was quite fed up when I arrived home from school – the fact that the treatment hadn't worked. I think David Cunningham was disappointed as well. The liver is such a strong organ. I get down but I still feel optimistic after a fairly short while. This is due to Lourdes, I'm sure – the feeling of hope and optimism. There has got to be a reason for all this pain and grief – I just don't know what.

Saturday 20th

Funny, I can manage with Shaun now and I can envisage his actual death. What I can't come to terms with is his actual dying and how I will cope with the loneliness afterwards – I don't think I will stand the pain and suffering.

We have had a crisis this afternoon. Shaun had a severe pain in the tumour. I rang the Marsden and then a duty doctor came and gave him a pain-relieving injection and a prescription for morphine. This doctor had trained at the Sutton hospital and wished us all the best. Morphine to me means the beginning of the end. Anyway, Shaun became a lot more comfortable with the injection.

We were all meant to be going to Neil's 21st (Kathleen's son). Shaun was missed – Annie (Kathleen's sister) was upset – I came home after half an hour but Matt, Stuart and Jo stayed.

Shaun still in some pain when he moves.

Sunday 21st

'I don't know if I'm in Limbo or dying.' That was Shaun at 7.30 p.m. this evening. He was also feeling sorry for his Dad having had no-one to rock him (I was holding him and rocking him at the time). I tried to cheer him up although I feel really down. I rang the Marsden this morning and they advised increasing the morphine as we had had a bad night. It's making Shaun very woozy. Steve S., the Maidstone rugby player, was here at lunchtime. I'm afraid we were not very good company.

I drove out to Aylesford Priory tonight to go for a walk. Shaun knew I needed to go – and he knew why. What is the future for us? The Royal Marsden, London, has just won an award for the development of the drug David Cunningham told us about the other day – carbo-platin, a new drug for ovarian cancer. This is what Shaun starts with tomorrow.

Monday 22nd

I was very down this morning. I packed Shaun a bag because I didn't know whether they would keep him in.

Malcolm, a fellow teacher, was very good to me when I arrived at school. He could sense immediately that all was not right. Anyway, Shaun saw Dr Finlay; the pain, he thinks, is caused by internal bleeding and it should cure itself. Shaun has had the first lot of the new treatment and he has liquid morphine to take. He still feels not quite on this planet but the relief of knowing what caused the pain has brought us both comfort. Yesterday he certainly wasn't stoical; today the stoicism is coming back. Shaun has said that if he had had a gun yesterday he would have shot himself.

News later tonight from Nick that their car has been hit up the back.

Tuesday 23rd

Things are a little better although tonight I am depressed again. Met Michèal in Safeway and he asked how I really felt Shaun was doing. He knows what to say. The tears started because I cannot honestly see a long-term future for us.

Rang Carmel but she is on school journey.

Just a thought: before, any hug or cuddle – Shaun with his flat stomach, me with my shape – we seemed to fit. Now, like this evening, Shaun's stomach is so swollen and hard, the fit is too hard to make! His stomach is definitely in the way!

Alice says to watch the amount of lactolose Shaun is taking because it can cause diarrhoea.

When I went shopping today I bought some fillet steak. It will do for my birthday as we will be at The Hengist restaurant in Aylesford on Shaun's. But really, what does it matter that I celebrate my 46th birthday if I am to be a widow before my 47th? It might just as well be now. My future has been taken from me with this curse of a disease! Why us? Why do we deserve it? What have we done? The only thing to hang on to is that God takes the good young. There's a trite statement for you!

I am so tired. I just want to fall into bed but I can't yet. I know I must see to Shaun's medication first.

Tuesday 30th

Must be grateful in a way. We have had the warning since September 24th and therefore we have made the most of the time. Couldn't really have been closer if we'd tried. Must remember how much worse it must be for people whose relatives die suddenly. **I need to keep up hope!**

It's been a dreadful few days. Went to see Lizzie in her ballet on Saturday – very good – and then we spent Saturday evening with our long-standing friends, the M.s and the C.s, for a meal. I never thought we would get to London for this weekend but Shaun was determined even though he wasn't really well. We stayed at Mum and Dad's and we saw Joe Whooley saying Mass on Sunday morning in the little chapel.

It was Sunday night at 10.30 p.m. that everything went wrong again. Shaun was in great pain and at midnight an emergency doctor arrived who gave him heroin; this knocked out the pain somewhat. I saw Dr Gardner just after 8.15 a.m. on Monday morning to get more morphine and then I spoke to Dr Finlay at the Marsden. He said different people need different amounts of morphine – advised us to put it up to 20 ml a dose and then work out the pain control from there. Dr Gardner came in the afternoon; says the liver is swollen. Shaun has jaundice. Dr Gardner then spoke to Dr Finlay at the Marsden. As he was leaving I asked about the time-scale – how long did we have left? I said I had no idea – I knew we didn't have years, but was it months, weeks or days? He said a week or so at the most. That hurt – although deep down I knew, I didn't really want to know. I wanted to keep on hoping. What a burden to bear, knowing that I'm going to lose my husband, lover and friend in so short a time. Can't share this with Shaun – he is too ill to take it in, so for his sake back comes my cheerful face.

Kathleen's daughter, Teresa, and her father, Peter, called in this morning. I'm not going into school for a while. Tina, my aunt, said 500 children at her school prayed for Shaun today. Dr Gardner phoned at 8.00 p.m. to see how Shaun was. Sue fell on her nose at school today. Noreen told me that, yesterday, Mr Drew said that he knew where he would like his wife to be in our circumstances so I'm sure he is sympathetic to me having time off.

8

May 1–12 – Some Light amid the Darkness

Thursday 2nd

Shaun said that as he dozed on the bed he heard two voices speaking to him, but he didn't know who they were or what they were saying.

The district nurse came yesterday and asked lots of questions. She spoke about the nursing services available. Shaun is still jaundiced and uncomfortable with his stomach. He was a bit depressed last night – he says he doesn't know what is going on in his guts – or whether anything is working or not.

I alternate – I don't know what to think. Sometimes I think that if it is *absolutely* inevitable then let it be quick. I can't stand much more of this. Then I am afraid of just how the end will be – please God it will not be pain and suffering and haemorrhaging. I can't pray properly – I can only hold one-sided conversations. I say to God: 'Do you really want him more than I do?' Must keep to 'Thy will be done'.

Haven't really thought before how all this came about. Was there anything we could have done differently, to have stopped the cancer appearing in the first place – and why the hell did it have to go to the liver of all places? As Dr Gardner says, if the liver gets kicked it takes so much and then gets its own back. It has its own chemistry.

10.10 a.m.: Shaun's tummy is feeling a bit funny at the moment. He has gone back to bed. *I should be positive and not give up on the new treatment.*

Trouble this afternoon with piles caused by constipation – I collected suppositories and cream from the doctor. Tony S. arrived at 2.15 p.m.

and left at 7.30 p.m. About 4 o'clock Shaun just disappeared upstairs and stayed there for an hour and a half until the successful conclusion of the lactolose and suppositories combination. He had felt really bad – his legs couldn't use the stairs properly. He is like an old, old man. It must be crippling him mentally; he has always been so active throughout his life.

Rose brought me a marvellous basket of flowers for my birthday. Jo came to dinner – she is so caring and loving. I hope things work for them – she is good for me as well!

11.20 p.m.: I want a hug, but it hurts Shaun's stomach. I'm lonely already.

Friday 3rd

My birthday. Same age as Shaun for today – for the last time? I received many flowers. Teacher friend Rosemary, and Roger and Caroline, all said I deserved them. I don't feel I have the courage people seem to think I have.

Enormous bouquet from Shaun's firm, the Leadenhall, and more flowers from Rosemary.

Jim and Dick, from the Leadenhall, came to lunch today and Shaun seemed to buck up. Ann D. brought chocolate and a bottle of whisky for Shaun. Lionel called in tonight. He has spoken to The Hengist and fixed it for us to stay overnight if we want to. Shaun thought it was a lovely idea and it really was on the cards until we sat down to our meal tonight. Shaun fancied eating the Steak Diane and having a bottle of wine – but once the food was in front of him he felt ill. Dr Gardner had called in earlier and left a prescription for water tablets.

Malcolm is a comfort – he called in with lots of cards from school. Shaun told him he would buy him a pint sometime for being good to me.

I'm just thinking – the past has to move over to make way for the future.

Sunday 5th

My God, is it a testing time? Shaun's birthday yesterday. Jo, Matt and Stuart have promised us tickets for *Buddy*. Shaun's brother Terry and his wife, Geraldine, have brought us a framed photograph of ourselves taken at their 25th wedding anniversary. Shaun looks so well in it!

He really is so weak – he gets to the bottom of the garden just once a day and that's virtually it, apart from going upstairs. Dr Gardner came yesterday to wish him Happy Birthday.

Jo was here for lunch today and met Terry and Geraldine. Michàel came this morning and Fr Chris brought Shaun communion this afternoon. This waiting is really difficult. It hurts – seeing Shaun as he is and knowing what he should be like. He can't walk properly; he is thin. I now hope for his sake that the end is quick – to be honest, it will be better for all of us. The poor man is not my Shaun any more.

Mike rang yesterday from Australia and I know that he is upset.

This morning Shaun rang the Marsden but they said this tiredness was to be completely expected.

· I think of Joe-Joe, my grandfather, and how irritable he got with Nanna, and I remember understanding that he didn't mean it – it was the cancer. That is why I am not worried when Shaun gets a little bit cross. Sometimes he is right – I do fuss. I can't help asking if he is alright – or wants something to eat or drink. I can easily forgive him. Life is cruel to do this to what was a very fit, healthy man.

11.15 p.m.: Shaun woke up on the settee and wanted to go to bed. I helped him to undress and put him to bed and he was asking for morphine – he cannot remember having the last dose only two hours ago. Anyway, I have reassured him and I think I'll take the next dose up after three hours in total.

1.30 a.m.: Just checked. Shaun hasn't moved. Asleep on his back – mouth open. The man in my bed is dying. When Shaun speaks, his words are slurred; it is as though he is constantly drunk – but without the happy feelings.

I feel like an empty shell. If you opened me up I would be empty. I have given everything.

Tina has written to Knock – a shrine in Ireland. It would mean a trip on the Jumbulance, but I know we will never make it.

Monday 6th

'Everyone's suffering in a certain way.' Shaun said that this morning at about 9.00 a.m. He says he doesn't know what is wrong with him. He was near to tears as I held him for a while. He didn't like me seeing him like it. Last night I woke him at 12.15 a.m. for his morphine and he said, 'Why are you looking at me like that? You look as though I'm going to pop off at any moment.' It threw me – all I could say was, 'Now I know you're not.'

He is very conscious that he isn't forming his words properly; he says his jaw won't open completely.

Nick, Sue, Lizzie, Mum and Dad were down for a few hours this afternoon. Mum and Dad are obviously suffering because of all this and I haven't the real strength to help them.

Jo is a tower of strength – she has been here and this evening she came and sat with me for a talk. She is strong, yet she and Matt think I am brave – I have to keep an 'outside' face for people. She has told Matt that he can lean on her as I lean on him. Thank God, He has given her to us. Shaun came and sat with us in the front room for a change of scene – and then Matt joined us. I think Shaun has become more alert as the day got older. We joked that we needed to keep his eyelids open with matchsticks because although he was listening and sometimes joining in, he couldn't keep his eyes open.

Going back to this morning, it took nearly an hour for me to bath him and apply various creams and suppositories. The piles were bleeding but Shaun did not realise.

Tuesday 7th

I waited up until 12.15 a.m. to give Shaun his morphine and he was good. I don't think he was totally conscious but I was very satisfied. It was something he had wanted to do, even though I don't think my whole man was there.

This morning the car wouldn't start and Shaun is not too lucid for periods. He has trouble with the piles bleeding and it is bothering him. 'I had better go to the doctor's,' he said. I have phoned to ask the doctor to call.

I went back to bed with him this morning at 8.30 a.m. but Florrie, Shaun's mother, phoned an hour later. She says she wants to come on the coach. I told her to talk to Shaun's brother Terry. Terry rang later. Shaun tried to get up but he is so tired – he asked what day it was and when I told him, 'Tuesday', he said, 'Oh God, this could go on another week.'

2.30 p.m.: I feel trapped. Shaun is still in bed; I'm waiting for the doctor and I can't settle. I'm just pacing from room to room.

Dr Gardner has prescribed some complete food drinks – very

expensive and I ran down to the local chemist to get them but they haven't got them until tomorrow. I bought some branded liquid food and Shaun has had one and a half glasses. The doctor told Shaun he was doubly blessed, what with his tummy and his piles but they aren't to cause us worry – they are varicose veins really. Shaun got up at about 5.00 p.m. today – the latest ever. This evening he sat in the front room with me. He was comfortable and said he could be quite happy if things finished like this. I told him that if he was happy with that then I would be happy for him.

Chris, our mechanic friend, couldn't fix the car – coming again tomorrow. I feel more relaxed and optimistic tonight – funny thing is I don't know why.

Wednesday 8th

Phone calls and visitors. Mum E., Mum and Dad and Teresa called in. She is going to collect the prescription.

Well, I did it. I rang the Marsden and spoke to David Cunningham. He says there would be no point in going tomorrow. The last time he had seen Shaun the liver had enlarged a lot and was now completely resistant to the treatment. He was very sorry but thought that Shaun had had a quality to his life. They have tried their best I know, I should think that they are upset. Mary, the nurse, came and spoke about various options with regard to hospitalisation, nursing care, etc. She agrees with me, though, that home is best if at all possible. She brought a bottle and mentioned commodes, bath boards, etc.

Shaun has had a bath – it takes a while but we manage somehow. Terry phoned back (I had phoned him this morning); he had had to leave the office and walk for a while. I asked him to bring his Mum down tomorrow. He asked when I was going to talk to Shaun. I'm not sure what he meant – then he mentioned priests.

Dr Gardner called in and then our great friend Jim T. arrived from Scotland. I couldn't put him off as he had come such a long way yet I knew it would hurt him to see Shaun. As he was going he asked how things really were (I thought he had realised) and I upset him when I said that I didn't honestly think we had long left together. I wish in a way that I hadn't told him – yet he would have found out the truth anyhow. I might write him a quick letter. I actually managed to nip up to the shop while he was here. And Shaun had managed to get down to the apple tree at the bottom of our garden with Jim. He does like it down the end of his garden. I shall always remember Shaun sitting on the low branch of that tree just surveying his own garden.

Chris couldn't fix the car – probably the starter motor; will come again tomorrow.

Shaun has more or less slept all the time since Jim left, first on the settee and then at about 7.00 p.m. he went to the loo and then straight to bed. He said, 'I've got to wake up otherwise I won't get my strength back.' His speech wanders quite a bit. I undressed him at 9.00 p.m. He says I am making him a walking zombie – he's right I suppose, although not walking.

It's like a full circle – babyhood, growing up, adulthood, back to babyhood.

Thursday 9th

The washing of both body and soul. Ascension Day. Michèal has just anointed Shaun and given us both communion.

Harry, a friend who was strongly connected with Maidstone Rugby Club, called but did not see Shaun. He left in tears. Lionel phoned from Stockport. Dr Gardner plus Mary, the nurse, have both been.

Terry and Florrie arrived in the afternoon. I took them up to see Shaun and after five minutes he had had enough. He said he would have a sleep and then come down. He did try to get up – he insisted on getting dressed but didn't have any strength to do it, so somehow I managed it, helped him down the stairs and on to the settee. He fell asleep almost at once. He is so very yellow now – I know Terry and Florrie are upset.

Alf J., another friend through rugby, on the phone in tears – said that Jim T. had been very cut up.

Chris finally fixed the car – Michèal came back with a bottle of sherry for me and a begonia plant. He stayed to tea although, of course, Shaun was neither up nor eating. Shaun was mentioned in Mass this morning. Prayers were said for him.

Paul E., a very great friend through rugby, in tears on the phone.

Janet, a teacher from school, arrived with a Mass card this evening. She offered me her car if Chris cannot fix mine.

Dave and Mary M. and Pat C. have phoned tonight. Shaun is so popular and loved – no wonder God wants him early. Judy P., a peripatetic teacher from school, phoned and offered me a safe haven – somewhere I can just go and sit for a while. How lovely of her.

Apparently Ed and Sister Mary from St Simon Stock School want to take us out for a meal. Too late I know. They told Michèal that Shaun was the life and soul of the party in Lourdes – and he was! **11.10 p.m.**: I hear Shaun's voice: 'She!' I run upstairs. 'Say I'll ring back – I don't know who he is!' Shaun is dreaming – but who *is* calling him?? Rang Terry. He has spoken to cousin Brian, and relatives in Devon and Ireland. Brian is upset.

Is That It Now?

Friday 10th

I feel tired and down today. Stuart has stayed home. It takes longer to get Shaun awake enough to take the tablets now. A new nurse came today – Iris – talked about attendance allowance for those caring for someone as ill as Shaun. Ed phoned – wanted to take us both out to lunch next week, but of course it won't be possible. He is going to call in later.

Tina has phoned during her (late!) lunch hour from school. Every time I disturb Shaun he says: 'Is that it now?' He hasn't asked the time yet today which is something he had been constantly doing.

Commode arrived.

'Dad is there in little bits – normal self for a bit – and then he kind of changes.' Stuart said this this afternoon.

Ed and Sister Mary arrived just as Dr Gardner was leaving. He doesn't think it will be much longer than the weekend. Today has been hard – it is increasingly difficult to get Shaun to take the medication. He is fighting me off all the way. I have to smile – he pulled his fist back and said, 'I'll punch you!' His arm was going any place – he just does not have the control. He has not asked the time at all today. I think that is significant. He doesn't really comprehend anything.

Mr Drew arrived just after Ed left. He was very good – we talked about the future.

Peter C., Kathleen's husband, came up to see Shaun. Matt and Jo came home instead of going to a show in London. I appreciate that. Rose came. Ready-call nurse came to help me with the 8.00 p.m. medication. We needed two of us. Nice lady. Another two are coming at midnight. I am so weary.

11.00 p.m.: Shaun struggles as I try to get his legs back on the bed

after we had managed with the bottle. 'Is that it now?' he keeps saying.
He is so weary. Not my strong Shaun at all.

A Gift From God

Saturday 11th

I did not write this until the following Tuesday – there was obviously
no time. But events are still sharp in my mind.

Two nurses came at midnight and between the three of us we
managed to get the morphine into Shaun. I set the alarm for 3.40 a.m.
as they said they would be back at approximately 4 o'clock. It was
tougher to administer the dose this time – one of the nurses had to
kneel up on the bed behind Shaun, pushing him into a sitting position
so that we could get the medicine down his throat. By this time Shaun
was not aware of anything. He just wanted to be left in peace I suppose
and I wish it could have been possible, but I knew that without the
morphine he would have been in terrible pain.

After they left, I lay down on the bed beside Shaun. I started to
sleep but although I could shut off the nose of his very loud breathing,
he seemed all of a sudden to be in mental torment. He was back in his
childhood and calling out in an anguished way. It wasn't until I felt
his hand on my cheek and the smell that I realised what had happened.
It was really hard to wash and clean. Shaun was fighting all the way,
although he wasn't conscious and certainly did not know it was me.
Funny, although his body was so thin and weak, he had a lot of
strength still. However, I couldn't involve either of the boys in something so basic as this, so I had to cope. I also knew that I wouldn't get
a nurse at 8.00 a.m. as it was the change-over time. I woke Matt up
when it was time and between us we tried to give Shaun the morphine
but we just couldn't do it. He was resisting so strongly, it was impossible. I phoned Dr Gardner and he was here by 8.30 a.m., and gave
Shaun an injection of morphine. Later on the nurses fixed up a syringe
driver – the same type of pump which had administered Shaun's
chemotherapy, only this time it was put into his shoulder. It was
now Saturday. The boys were terrific – they fielded all visitors and
telephone calls.

There was one really hectic time mid-morning. Dr Gardner had
arrived back and two nurses were also here. One of the nurses was
talking to Shaun but of course there was no way he was taking any-

thing in – he just wasn't with us. She kept saying she wanted to give him a wash, even though I kept telling her that I had been through all that in the early hours of the morning. She kept trying to turn him on his side, but she didn't have any success. She was concerned about bed sores she said. The nurses just didn't seem to realise how close Shaun was to God – and to death. As if bed sores were going to matter now! Inwardly I was screaming – why can't they leave him in peace and stop pulling him around? I *knew* this was to be his last day. He was going to leave us for better things later. Let him die in peace. Eventually they managed to prop him up on five pillows, on my side of the bed. I remember being very cross about that – why was Shaun going to die on my side of the bed? Oddly enough, it has been a great comfort to me since. When I get into bed at night now, it is not as though I have to reach out to an empty space, but rather that Shaun is right there with me, on my side. Sometimes I can almost feel him. I hope that feeling lasts.

A lovely nurse came in the afternoon – Lyn L. As she was going off duty she left me her home phone number – something she always warns her nurses against.

Shaun was very restless. Calling out, still in his childhood, certainly not with us. Very loud breathing, and mental anguish still. At one point both Matt and I held him and told him that it was alright for him to go. He was not aware that we were there. As he became more agitated I used Lyn L. number and she returned to *up* the dose of morphine. She quietly sat talking to me as Shaun seemed to settle down more; the anguish seemed to have subsided somewhat and he appeared to sleep, although every now and then he became a little restless. It was at this point that Fr Jim arrived and the boys let him through. He came and just sat with Shaun and I in the bedroom for a good hour. Obviously Shaun was not aware that he was there but I certainly appreciated it. I wish in a way that Fr Jim had been there later as well so that he could have witnessed what we did. He said later that it had been a privilege for him to have been there.

All I could do now for Shaun really was to wet his lips occasionally with water. He was incapable of eating or drinking and he was plagued with these terrible hiccups which looked as though they hurt, though I don't suppose they did. I was told that they were due to the movement of the diaphragm.

In the early evening Annie came in, offering to nurse Shaun for me, but there was no way I was giving up now. I had come this far; I would see it through. In fact I didn't feel tired any more; yet I hadn't slept properly for weeks and had certainly had very little sleep over the past 48 hours. Some inner strength must keep you going.

Teresa and her sister-in-law Lyn arrived and I told Matt and Jo to go out for an hour. They had had no respite either. The three of us women sat round the bed, with a drink in our hands, holding Shaun's hands and trying to help him with the terrible hiccups which kept jolting him. When Matt came back later, he said that he always knew that women were the strongest.

Later on, after Teresa and Lyn had gone, Dr Hart, the doctor on duty, arrived to see how things were. After he left, I had a few mouthfuls of food, which tasted like sawdust, and then suddenly Shaun's breathing changed. I called the boys, feeling slightly apprehensive because I wasn't sure how the end would be – would it be violent and bloody, or would it be peaceful? Anyway, the boys had a right to be there if they wished and at this stage I thought that we probably only had a few minutes left. Instead, we had over an hour of real peace. We were blessed; we knew that They were talking to Shaun and occasionally through Shaun's muttered conversations we could clearly hear what he said. This was not a figment of my imagination – all three of us heard the same things and we were sitting in different positions around the bed. At one point Shaun said, 'Am I coming back?' Then, we heard him say a little later, 'I'll go over here, then.'

Shaun looked so peaceful, propped up on the pillows, resting on one elbow, with his eyes open for the first time in more than 24 hours, just looking upwards into the distance. I felt I couldn't say anything to him for fear of interrupting this lovely conversation he was having – it seemed to bring him great peace. I just held his hand – I would have been intruding on something so very personal and private to him, yet in a way, probably without knowing it, he **was** sharing it with us. At one point Matt had held his other hand and said, 'I love you, Dad' and Shaun had whispered a reply – again, one that we all heard – 'I love you all too.'

About 20 minutes before he finally died, Shaun's face suddenly lit up; he had the look that a person has on their face when they suddenly see someone they haven't seen for years. How do you describe it – joy, happiness and recognition all rolled into one? His voice also held all three of these emotions as he said, 'Our Father,' and then, 'Hail Mary.' The tone of voice held wonderment, reverence and love. We all heard this part of the conversation. We looked at each other and repeated what Shaun had said. I don't think any of us could quite believe it – a miracle, and a gift from God to us. We *knew* then that

Shaun was in Heaven, even though he breathed on, very shallowly for another 20 minutes. We are really blessed to have witnessed this. No-one can ever remove these memories from any of us. It is the legacy left to us which will hold us for ever.

Jo was marvellous. The poor girl was shattered, yet as the three of us came downstairs she was there to give us all a hug; she put the kettle on to make the tea and she poured the brandy. We telephoned Dr Hart. He warned us of the dangers of drinking too much tea and coffee, as we sat there with mugs in our hands. He also said to be prepared for people to ignore us as they often don't know what to say. In fact, that has only happened once – the reverse has more often been true.

Matt rang the undertakers when Dr Hart left and we had an hour to wait. I suddenly got very afraid of seeing them. I did not want to see Shaun removed from our house, even though I knew he wasn't in that poor, sick body any more. Jo dealt with it all, while the boys and I sat in the back room talking about anything to take our minds off of what was happening upstairs.

Matt helped me to change our bed; Jo insisted on the sleeping bag on the settee and we all tried to sleep for a little while. After all it was 4.30 a.m. I think I must have slept a little, because, although I had phoned Terry while waiting for the undertakers, I had many more phone calls to make early in the morning.

9

May 12–31 – Somehow
Buoyed up amid the Grief

Sunday 12th

I rang the presbytery early and Michèal said he would come after saying Mass at Preston Hall. In fact, he came straight away; Jo was still in the sleeping bag, although awake, and this was the first time she had met him. After he left, Peter and Teresa came, and later Sabine, an ex-teacher friend, and her husband Terry, called in – the news had spread fast. Terry and Geraldine arrived at lunchtime, and so did Nick, Sue, Mum and Dad. It was a most peculiar feeling – everything was functioning, as though this was perfectly normal. Sister Kathleen, a teacher at school, and Sister Eileen, the Parish Sister, arrived with another Mass card. Things hadn't hit us; we were on automatic pilot.

Matt and I went down to 6.00 p.m. Mass – strange, really, when you think of it afterwards, but it was something we wanted to do. Michèal said he hadn't expected us but I am pleased we went. I shall never forget the reaction of Yvonne, a friend, when it was announced from the pulpit that Shaun had died that morning.

After we came home, Michèal came again to say that he and Fr Jim had decided that we could use the presbytery after the funeral. I was overwhelmed – that was such a big kindness – something they had never done before. Michèal persuaded us to go over to the club for a drink with the C.s. I didn't feel right about it, until he asked what Shaun would have wanted and what Shaun would have done. I suppose I was still functioning on automatic pilot; in fact I now know I was, although at the time everything seemed normal. Shock, I suppose. I slept fully that night – the first time in weeks.

Letters

Monday 13th

I was woken early by the postman who brought a whole stack of cards and letters. Stuart couldn't walk when he woke up – he had hurt his knee yesterday but I hadn't taken much notice. Anyway, I took him to casualty, praying that he hadn't broken any bones again. I asked the woman the waiting time, as, I told her, I had to go and collect my husband's death certificate. She must have thought what a hard, cold bitch I was – to speak like that while showing little or no emotion – but again I suppose it is the shock that in a way protects you and shields you. We were pushed to the front of the queue, anyway, and Stuart had strained the ligaments in his knee. When we arrived home, Terry was waiting to take me to the undertakers, etc. Matt came as well and we sorted out the details of the funeral for the following Monday. We were lucky enough to be able to choose our double plot – right in front of Kathleen; this has given us and the C.s a little comfort. Afterwards we went to the Registry Office to collect the death certificate. I found the word *widow* upsetting. I had also been upset earlier while choosing the coffin. It isn't something you are prepared for doing really. We left the Registry Office and went up to look at the plot in the cemetery – a very nice place; Terry thought it was peaceful.

Tina and Peter, my aunt and uncle, brought Mum and Dad down at about 5.00 p.m. and friends from school, Noreen and Tricia, arrived from school with more Mass cards.

Tuesday 14th

This morning, again waking up early for the postman, I felt very organised. Actually, I looked forward to the postman coming – so many lovely and varied memories of Shaun coming from people. I would make a cup of tea and then go back upstairs and read them all. They really sustained me. I made lots of phone calls in a very businesslike way – bank, insurance, gas, and electricity board . . . Again, I suppose it was a question of functioning on automatic pilot.

In the evening, I took Lionel and Elizabeth down to the church so that Lionel could run through the hymns we had chosen on the organ. He had never heard any of them, but he did remarkably well. Fr Chris joined us later and sang them for us. We went into the presbytery afterwards and had a very nice conversational evening with Fr Jim over a bottle of wine. Really, the last few days have been so hard that this was a nice break. As long as I can keep busy and think that what I am doing is useful then I am alright. I am spending a lot of time planning the funeral service: I do not want it to be morbid or gloomy if I can possibly help it: I want it to be a celebration of Shaun's life – I know he wouldn't have wanted everyone weeping and wailing.

More Letters

Wednesday 15th

Today, after reading all my post – a lovely feeling, really (Shaun would be most embarrassed to know how much he meant to people) – I finalised the funeral service. In the evening Matt, Stuart, Jo and I went to The Wheelers, where Michàel joined us later. Paul and Jim, licencees of The Wheelers, had not heard of Shaun's death, and Paula just left the bar, very upset. Michèal came back with us where we watched the wedding video. We didn't go to bed until 1.50 a.m., slightly the worse for wear.

Thursday 16th

Have been very tired and down today. I bought a skirt and blouse for next Monday. Old friends Ruby and Frank arrived about 4.45 p.m. – a nice surprise – I didn't know they were coming.

I spoke to Shaun's aunt, Ann, in Chichester, and later to Terry B. from the teaching profession. He is upset that he now will not be able to make the funeral. I told him not to worry. I have a feeling that there will be lots of people in the church on Monday.

Friday 17th

Duncan, my cousin, arrived in the evening with young Luke. He knows what I am going through and it was nice to see him. Duncan will not be able to make the funeral as he has a job to start on Monday, but he and Lesley are coming down on Sunday evening when Shaun's body will be taken into church.

After he had gone, I felt miserable. Tiredness, I expect. Shaun would never have expected so much interest, I think. To date I have received 183 cards, Mass cards and letters. The postman has had to knock every morning – too many to put through the letter box. Today he actually asked me whether Shaun had died. He said that on Monday he just thought there was an important birthday, but as the days went on he couldn't help noticing that all the letters and cards were addressed to me and the boys. I find great comfort in them. I talk to Shaun's photo often. I miss him so much. I keep expecting him back, really. Hope I can keep strong – if it wasn't for the boys . . . How do people carry on without their loved one?

Saturday 18th

Another sad day. Lionel came in the morning. Nick, Sue and Lizzie came in the afternoon. Josephine arrived with the girls. She brought a big cake. Spurs won the cup. After they had gone, I was very sad. I cried all over Matt down the end of the garden, and I upset him; which meant that Jo then had to comfort him. I must be careful. Funny how each day is different. Yesterday, for part of the day, I felt good – positive – kept talking to Shaun and smiling. It has been an unreal week.

A Green Balloon

Sunday 19th

Lots of people came to the 6.00 p.m. Mass tonight. Terry and Geraldine brought Florrie while Dave and Mary brought Mum and Dad. Tina and Peter, Duncan and Lesley also came. Fr Chris said Mass, and then at 7.00 p.m. when Mass had finished, Shaun's body was brought into church. Fr Chris was kneeling in front of the coffin saying the Glorious Mysteries of the rosary, when all of a sudden this green balloon with the word 'Joy' painted on it came drifting slowly down the aisle. I had noticed it during Mass; it was stuck up on the ceiling, but I hadn't thought a lot about it.

There had been a children's Mass this morning and they had all held balloons with the gifts of the Holy Spirit written on them. One of the children had obviously let this particular green one go. Anyway, this balloon floated slowly to the altar, and hovered in mid-air. As Matt said, it was the Irish green. It was just as though Shaun was saying to us, 'I'm alright' . . . Almost as though he were there. Some people thought it was a custom and we had arranged it – but the balloon lifted us all – it was so symbolic. I rang Nick and Sue to tell them and when they arrived with their wreath they had inserted a green balloon with the word 'Joy' painted on it. Marvellous!

Many People, Many Happy Memories

Monday 20th

Nervous really at the start – what could go wrong? I had tried so hard to cover every contingency. Woken up at 6.55 a.m. by flowers from Tony and Theresa (my mother's cousins) – delivered by brown dormobile. Michèal came to collect the orange-juice, etc. and then I got a phone call from the undertakers. Too many flowers!

The Irish group arrived with Terry and then Mum and Dad, Nick and Sue and then the Devon group with Geraldine.

The Mass was beautiful – it couldn't have been better. Standing room only in the church. Fr Jim spoke *so* well about Shaun – it *must* have touched everyone's hearts. Lionel played the organ superbly and the St Simon Stock choir were marvellous. It was a real celebration of Shaun's life. I know he's gone and this day was good, but I still expect him to come back – it is as though he is away on a trip.

I have never seen so many people at a cemetery, or so many floral tributes – 83 in total.

I wasn't really sad as the coffin was lowered so deeply – the essence of the man was not in that coffin, Shaun was not in there really – we have so much proof. All I could think of was that Shaun would have said: 'What good soil!' I'm not being blasphemous or disrespectful.

It was really good to have the presbytery – so many people with so many good memories of Shaun, and enough food and drink for all. The family came home afterwards, plus Roger and Delyth, and then we went with Terry, Geraldine, Florrie, Jo and Jo's mother Ann, to the Running Horse for a meal.

Wednesday 22nd

Was apprehensive – Matt back to work and Stuart back to school. I took chocolates in for the choir.

Went to the solicitors. Things should be alright; then I met Alice for coffee.

Mike phoned from Perth. Sunday 12th May had been Mother's Day out there and the first baby born entered the world at 2.15 a.m., and was named Shaun! Mike has asked us to spend Christmas out there. I don't think I can.

Teachers Janet and Catherine arrived from school with peaches, strawberries, pineapple, oranges and cream!

Spoke to both Janet and Carmel – they are full of the funeral.

Today I feel that Shaun is just around the corner. He has to wait for me until the boys are settled and then – God willing – I can join him.

Thursday 23rd

Not a good day today. Took some of Shaun's clothes to the Cancer Research shop, went shopping and planted some seedlings. Fergus W. brought me a book by Graham Clarke – a local artist we admire. Nigel R., who had supplied the drink for the funeral, collected what remained; Frances came back from Canada, very upset. I feel down. Wrote some letters today – another reason for being down I suppose. I really miss Shaun; I want to hold him and him to hold me. God it is hard. I loved – love – him so much. I want him here with me now! How do people cope? I sometimes don't think I can.

Had a dream last night and Shaun – in his blue suit – was standing just around the corner but I couldn't see his face. Still nice comments coming about Shaun. Theresa S., a friend from my school days in Charlton, wrote to say you could feel the love for Shaun shine out at the Mass. Kashmiro remembers Shaun writing on her leaving card, 'Life is Magic'. What a beautiful thought that he actually thought that!

Saturday 25th

Mixed day today. Went to 10.00 a.m. Mass – it was for Shaun. Sr Eileen and Sr Mary were there. I went back to 6.00 p.m. this evening with Stuart. More people offering their condolences. I never really know how to reply. Jo and Matt have gone for a meal this evening. Frances' daughter, Josephine, came this afternoon; new furniture arrived and the chair is not right!

Yesterday was not a bad day. Took cream cakes in for the teaching staff – went to assembly and then went back again in the afternoon for 'The Clothes Show', a small school concert. Have spoken to my class – I need to get back. Fr Jim came at 7.00 p.m. and spent two very nice hours. I know I didn't stop talking but he was very patient with me. As he left, Shelagh O., husband Bobby and their son Christopher arrived – with three plants, chocolates and a card! Christopher had organised a collection in school. A pleasant evening – they stayed until 11.50 p.m.

Terry B. called this evening. He and his wife, Vicky, are coming to see me on Monday.

Funny, can't seem to write my feelings properly any more. All I seem to be doing is putting down facts, not feelings. My logical side knows where Shaun is and that he is at peace and must be so happy – his reward for having been such a nice person – but my other side cries out for hugs and kisses and wanting to hold him near. I miss him so much – I keep saying he is waiting for just an interval – how long is that interval to be? I tell Shaun that I will stay until the boys are settled and old enough – but will God let me go to him then?

I am weary of this life but obviously God knows I am not worthy yet to go to the next.

Don't get me wrong – people are marvellous – very supportive. But **nobody** can know exactly how I feel – no-one can get inside me to know, except God. It still seems so unreal – wrong to ask, I know – but why do I deserve it? People keep saying I'm brave, but by God I'm not.

Sunday 26th

Sometimes I feel physically sick, I miss him so. Mum and Dad were down today. They are sad, too. Hank and Anne called in for a little while this morning. Geraldine's sister, Rita, is in hospital.

I break down heavily when I'm on my own. I wish for the end of the world so that we can all be reunited. I must stop being like this – I have to get used to it – but I hurt.

Tuesday 28th

A very nice evening. Geraldine arrived at about 4.30 p.m. and we went to St Peter's at Bearsted for Mass. Lovely church – so peaceful – many references to Shaun throughout the Mass, and the readings and sermon were all about having a smile on your face; and Fr Chris was saying how hard it was to do all the time. Lovely. Noreen and husband Eddie, Mary and Steve, Tricia, Janet and family and former school secretary Irena, and husband Ted were all there. We went upstairs afterwards for coffee and we all brought flowers home. Met Breda for the first time – mother of five including Roisin, who was in the group who went to the cinema with Stuart today. The T.s are really brave. I wasn't this morning – phoned Mícheal and he came straight away. I can cry with him – it hurts. I still feel that maybe I will wake up from this nightmare.

I am worried about Matt – he is so tired and has been suffering since Shaun died. Pauline came at lunchtime and Irena this afternoon.

Yesterday I was bad. St Francis Teacher Margaret C., Terry, Vicky and Terry B.'s son, Jonathan came. In the evening Jo, Matt, Stuart and I played Scrabble.

'Yes' to Australia

Friday 31st

The last day of a tumultuous month. Stuart finally signed off from the hospital. I have booked – and paid for – three tickets to Australia for Christmas. I have changed my mind and feel it would be much better to be there at Christmas rather than here. I pray to God that Shaun agrees with what I have done.

Stuart and I went to the cemetery and threw away the dead flowers. Still lots left, though. I shed a few tears there. Strange to think I have seen my final resting place. Stuart thinks I'm lucky – but he did say that he didn't want me to go yet – he doesn't much fancy moving house!

Had a marvellous letter from Pat C.: made me cry – but it was really good. I phoned him tonight – he said he started to write it in a hotel bedroom in York but got too upset. He then did something he doesn't normally do – went to the bar and had lots of glasses of port. He went back upstairs at 12.40 a.m. very much the worse for wear – and phoned Julie!

Dear Sheila.

Many years ago, Shaun and I were on an Easter Rugby tour in Southend – of all places – when I wanted to send a post-card. I was complaining that the selection on offer was dreadful, and Shaun became offended. 'So what?', he said. 'They won't worry about the card. It's the fact that you've remembered to write, that's what matters'. I remembered that when I started to scribble this note on headed notepaper and in hand-writing which nobody could possibly understand. So I screwed it up, as he would have wanted, and reached for the W. H. Smith's paper and elderly typewriter. So . . .

Dear Sheila,

On the evening of Shaun's funeral, Dave, Fin and I sat in the Royal Oak and talked about him. We remembered only the good days; playing, laughing and drinking with him. Time was when we couldn't accept that he was a far, far better player than we could ever hope to be. I remember playing with him down at Esher, soon after he took up the game. He scored three tries that day. 'That's all very well', I said, 'but the game's not as easy as you seem to think'. 'You're probably right', he said. 'By the way, how many did *you* score today?' Of course, he went on to become the kind of player that we should all have wanted to be, but he never lost that strange sense of wonder at his own talent. In truth, we were far more annoyed by his modesty than by his extraordinary ability.

Some of us saw Shaun as the slim, muscular fellow with the long blond hair and wiggling shoulders that seemed to have a mind of their own. Physically and technically he could have made it to the top, but he was cursed by a fatal modesty. And it was that modesty which made us love him.

Shaun never had the remotest idea of his own value; not in Rugby and not in life. For some strange reason, he thought he'd cracked it by having a wife whom he adored and sons of whom he was justly proud. And those of us who have been blessed with similar fortune could only agree with his reasoning.

So Dave, Fin and I sat in the bar, took our cue from that wonderful Mass and refused to mourn a friend who had simply refused to grow old. Yet still we remembered how much we had lost. I shall be eternally grateful that I shared an evening with him just before the end, and far more grateful that I knew him in the good days when his life was an open book.

I hope you won't mind me writing like this, even though I can hear Shaun saying: 'Leave off, Collins'. But I did want to tell you how much he meant to us and how much we admired the example which you set at the Requiem Mass. Please God your faith will continue to sustain you through your grief. And please God we shall all continue to celebrate his short and beautiful life. God rest him.

With love & sympathy,

Pat

P.S. I've just read through this & I'm afraid it's a bit rambling. I so hope you won't be offended, and that you'll accept that I meant well.

It is a nice thought that Shaun can see *all* of his friends now – he can look down on them all at the same time. I bet he is having a few smiles. I have lost a beautiful man – people's memories written in these letters show that I wasn't just looking at him through rose-coloured glasses.

It often feels as though Shaun is away on tour – he will return. I can at times feel his arms around me – but they don't hug quite hard enough. Shaun, if you're listening, hug me hard!

10

Thank God May is Over

Saturday 1st

I used to like May, what with it having both our birthdays.

Matt and Jo took Stuart to the gym and I bought two water-colours for the priests. Went to see Sister Kathleen and she let slip that Michèal was leaving. I phoned him and he came round. Three weeks and he'll be off to St Winifred's at Wimbledon. Anyway, I gave him one of the paintings – he made me write on the back and date it. I shall miss him – and Mum and Dad, Terry, Nick and Sue all feel the same.

Terry is making a cross to mark the grave for me.

Jo has bought me strawberries this week.

Phoned Mike in Australia. Shed yet more tears today – I wish it were five years gone and I could go.

Nice letter from David Cunningham.

10.10 p.m.: Have just come back from the School Governors' Meeting. I think it was the right decision to go back to school. Had flowers and chocolates from some of the children. I was fine Monday while in the classroom – until I got in the car at 4.00 p.m. Then the tears flowed.

Monday and Tuesday evenings I spent doing reports.

Went to Mass twice on Tuesday and again at lunchtime today. And tomorrow! Sister Eileen talked to me and that started me off. She says it is good to cry.

Thursday 6th

Terry and Geraldine have been tonight. Terry has made a beautiful cross for Shaun's grave. We took it up and it looks lovely. Went to The Wheelers for a couple of hours and then home for dinner. Geraldine talked about my nephew Philip's friend, Adam, who had died tragically some time ago. Went to Mass again at lunchtime. Met Irena and Ted.

Still feel Shaun is on tour.

Was given a lovely plant by Nicola W. – a girl in my class.

Friday 7th

Paid the funeral bill at lunchtime and borrowed a brochure for head-stones. Will probably be well over £1000 by the time I have that verse put on it.

Fr Jim is talking about us all going to Brighton to gain ideas for St Francis from a school layout there – and have a meal as well.

Mrs A., a parent, was nice tonight – wanted me to visit.

Mary and Steve came into school with beautiful flowers. Told Mary that I had written them a letter but hadn't been able to bring myself to post it. I hope things go well for her – she has her last chemotherapy on Monday. I want to see more of them. Steve says that Mary keeps him going. I believe that – it must be so hard for him.

Jo and Matt set off for Sevenoaks in my car. Phoned me from Borough Green – car broken down. Jo has just phoned now (10.40 p.m.). They are back at the Walnut Tree – AA rescue. Not sure yet what is wrong.

I wonder how much time I still have to endure? That is how it feels at the moment. It could be 30 years! How on earth do you cope with such a span of loneliness? Real purgatory. I'm trying to tell people that they must cheer when I go. I still can't really believe that Shaun has gone. I don't *want* to believe it. I need him – here – now – with me. Why has it happened?

Saturday 8th

A quote: 'I never feel angry with God. He gives you the cross you can bear.' I *don't* feel angry with God. He really gives me the strength to go on. I don't know, though, that I can bear the cross. Nick, Sue and Lizzie were down tonight. We went to 6.00 p.m. Mass and then up to the cemetery. I think I will settle for a dark grey headstone; with the poem and a shamrock. We had a nice evening. Nick is having Shaun's blazer.

Tried to tidy the greenhouse a bit this afternoon.

The cemetery is not daft exactly (to go there, I mean) but I can't think of Shaun being in there – I know he isn't. It is just a memorial, a marker – a quiet, peaceful place – to recall memories, to talk, to shed tears (why??). I can't accept that he is there. He is just around the corner, waiting, for an interval. How long must the interval be? My purgatory will probably last until I'm 90! Now is the one time I wish I could see into the future. So that I could make plans for my going.

Something to look forward to. Shaun saying, 'I'll go over there, then.' I know he is on the right hand side of God. Marvellous, uplifting feeling. I do think I was so lucky to have been part of, and married to, a saint for all those years.

Lourdes Reunion

Sunday 9th

A very emotional afternoon – Lourdes reunion. Peter H. was there. He is seeing Dr Smith at the Marsden and is now on the pump and a Hickman line, but a weekly one. Sixth formers Melanie and Kelly (helpers on the Lourdes trip), pilgrims Alison and Tamsin and Hilary, a nurse, were all there. Ann, a teacher friend, played for the Mass. Michèal anointed me and many others. Three of the hymns were the same as for Shaun's funeral, plus the Lourdes hymn. I really couldn't stop myself crying. It was so hard. Melanie gave the sermon – beautiful. There was Labie Siffré music among other tunes. She is going to send me a copy of the tape. The girls were emotional, too.

Talked to Ann about purgatory and the wish to pass through it. She told me about a friend of hers whose new-born baby had died shortly before Shaun. Ann comforted her by saying that she knew of a wonderful father who had now gone to take care of her. What a nice thought. She also mentioned Shelagh and Bobbie O. again and their belief that Shaun's 'brother' – someone who looked just like him – was sitting behind us at the funeral.

Matt, Jo and Stuart have gone to the Malta Inn – I would not be good company. They have come up trumps again with their work in the garden. Mum and Dad are back from France.

Quote from the Blackthorn Trust*: 'Being ill opens up new perspectives which were hidden within you.' Positive thinking came out of this programme. Shaun had this feeling without the Blackthorn Trust. He would have been an ideal helper.

Thought: Would Jesus have viewed life on earth as purgatory? I think probably so. Funny, we enter into life with hope, happiness and positive thoughts – but is it really so? No! Not when you go through what I have.

Teresa was saying this morning that Peter's reaction to Shaun's death was to thank God that his age was such that he didn't have as long to wait (to be reunited) as I did – going by the law of averages. Also he made a comment about the people who visited him – they were Kathleen's friends – because they don't come now. Even though he says he is not bothered, that is a sad reflection. I am guilty – I do not go down to see him. I used to go and sit with Kathleen on a Saturday afternoon – now I go to the cemetery. Where, of course, I can still talk to her.

Wednesday 12th

Obviously the last couple of days haven't been horrific otherwise I would have found time to write. Today was not good, though, at school.

Was meant to meet Elizabeth but we muddled up the times. Janet, Sue and Paul all phoned this evening. Spoke to Terry – really sobbed tonight. I am beginning to realise that maybe Shaun is not just away on tour – that maybe he really isn't going to come back.

Stuart surprised me – told me today that it is a month since Shaun died. Of course I was counting the four weeks to last Sunday, but he is right as well.

Being Strong

Mum and others have said it was a good job I was the strong one – I can cope. What they don't seem to realise is that I was only strong as part of a partnership. I am what Shaun made me and I suppose he was what I made him. A true partnership – no need to double up: we worked things between us. No wonder half of me is missing – is dead – and has gone, I think, forever. I need him to function as I did. Life in the future has got to be so different.

Thursday 13th

A better day today. I told Mr Drew that I wouldn't mind taking the middle class that nobody wanted.

Nice comments from Mrs E., a parent, today.

Went to sort out arrangements for the headstone.

Lionel came to collect various certificates and brought a whole folder of letters from brokers plus £600, collected at the Leadenhall, for the Royal Marsden. That makes over £900 so far. Marvellous really.

Michèal called in as well.

Sunday June 16th

Mini-market yesterday – an annual parish event. I worked at 'our stall' (the school's bottle stall) for a bit and won a bottle of rum. Matt won sherry and Jo won a can of beer. Went to the cemetery afterwards.

Today the four of us set off for Hank and Anne's and promptly came to a halt on the M25, eleven miles from home. We were towed home so it cost me lunch at the Bull plus attendant taxi fares. Chris has now been, and will bring a modulator tomorrow.

Phone calls from Julie and my Auntie June.

A thought: It is what we do with our lives which marks our place in the universe.

Another thought: When I wake each morning I should be grateful that I am one day nearer being with Shaun.

Wednesday 19th

12 o'clock midnight: Stupid isn't it? Probably this time last year it was hot and I didn't want it – but it is so chilly this year that I need to be cuddled. I've lost what was said on television about the weather, but I remember now: May 21st was hotter than any day since the beginning of the year. May 20th (the funeral) was really warm as well. Best of the year so far.

Stuart's open night tonight at St Simon Stock School. Everyone thinks he is great – I know he doesn't let us down.

Went out with Jenny, a teacher at St Simon Stock, last night.

Nigel, an ex-Maidstone rugby player, phoned tonight: a daughter! A week ago. Odile!

Thursday 20th

11.30 p.m.: Shaun knows I am practical. Is it practical at the age of 46 to do without cuddles, hugs and even physical love-making for the rest of my earthly life? Yet how can I get comfort? He isn't here – well, yes, he is spiritually – but not physically. I need that love and comfort. I don't suppose that is being practical – just human. I love Shaun so much – why has God taken him? Why can't I be with him for his cuddles? Total honesty – I miss the physical side – it was so good. I shouldn't really be putting all this in a diary – who might read it? But it *is* how I feel and that, I suppose, is human?

Sunday 23rd

Nick, Sue, Lizzie and Mum came down this afternoon. Dad is not very well. Shelagh and Pete took Stuart and me out for a meal yesterday. Stayed talking to Jo until 2.45 a.m.

Paul and Brenda came Friday – friends of ours through rugby. Had a nice evening.

10.05 p.m.: I have rung Sue and unloaded a lot of tears. I miss Shaun so much. How can I go on without him? When can I wake up from this terrible dream?

Thought: Emotions after you die must be different. Given that everything is perfect in Heaven, the people who've gone there can't possibly be missing those they've left behind otherwise they would be feeling like I do and that would be very sad and therefore not perfect. How does that work, then? If Shaun isn't feeling upset, then maybe he isn't missing me? It is a peculiar thought. **I miss him. I need him.** I don't want to go on. I haven't got the strength.

Wednesday 26th

Three nights of Parent-Teacher consultation evenings are over. Not been quite as bad as I thought. Parents have been very nice. Went to Noreen's last night. She knew I was down. It was a nice evening.

Had a letter from old acquaintance Den yesterday – he hadn't heard about Shaun. He said his wife Olwyn's death had come suddenly.

Letter this morning from Kelly – she felt Shaun's presence during her revising for her A levels. Wants a photo of us together. Martin, a broker friend of Shaun's, has sent my car insurance for free. I must write to him because I didn't expect it this year.

Saw Dr Gardner tonight. He will fix an appointment for me to see a dermatologist. He read between the lines very well – said Shaun would give me a kick up the backside if he knew how I was thinking. Dr Gardner knew why I was smoking so much and wouldn't force me to give it up at this stage. Called me a 'long-term project'. He was pleased we are going to Australia.

* The Blackthorn Trust. A charitable organisation set up to help the sick. People attend classes in art, gardening, handicrafts, etc., as a form of therapy. Staffed by volunteers.

Sunday 30th

Went to Mum and Dad's today. All four of us. A nice day. Saw Nick and Sue for half an hour. Nick was playing golf this afternoon but did badly!

Spoke to Ann (Jo's Mum, who lives in Milford Haven) tonight. She wants me to go down to Wales to stay with her and David after we break up for the school holidays. I went to the cemetery – headstone marker is in place.

Matt was in Oxford Fri/Sat. Enjoyed the Curry House! Stayed at Merton College.

Bet rang this morning. It's nice to hear from old friends.

Why do I pretend? I am not taking this well! I miss Shaun so much. Why did God do this to me? Was I really so complacent before that I needed to be given a shock? It is obviously something I have done. Shaun, after all, has got the richest reward – I have the punishment. And yet – God is not into the business of being evil. So what is it really? I don't think I am as strong as people think. I am not. I sob for him – no, for myself – because I need Shaun so much. I am just functioning mechanically. I need to be with him. Why did God need him at 47? Funny, with all the friends and acquaintances, who can I be totally honest with? Only God, I suppose. And then I get angry! I feel almost let down at times – and yet, without faith, how do people cope?

11

A Growing Sense of Loss

Tuesday 2nd

Fr Jim has just gone. Good of him to come. He said something: after the deaths of Kathleen and Shaun he felt it wasn't harsh – or the end – but rather a smooth moving on to another place, done very gently. Not a hard shut off, the end. He said it was the faith of the families and how they had coped. A very nice thought to ponder, that it was gently done. *And it was, really.* If I am totally honest I could not be mean enough to have Shaun back here with me as he was for the last week – that would be cruel. I would love to have him back as he was in Lourdes; even though he was suffering somewhat, he still smiled through it. What a strong man he was! What an example to everyone who knew him. No wonder he has got his early reward!

Thursday 4th

I'm tired I know and I'm on my own. And I'm pretending. What is the future?

Matt and Jo go off tomorrow for a well-deserved holiday in Ireland. Their future is in front of them. Mine has gone. What is left?

Lionel gave me a cuddle tonight. He doesn't like to see me down. I miss Shaun holding me so much. I would gladly and willingly give up all this 'silly money' now – I want him back!!! Impossible. Why? Shaun has the reward, I have the punishment. How do I get to the next plane? What do I have to do to be that good? Help me, show me, guide me.

Wrote to Melanie and Kelly. Great girls.

Saturday 6th

Went to the cemetery and as usual shed a few tears but I actually walked away with a spring in my step and a smile on my face. My man was not in there: the poor, tired, jaundiced body no doubt is, but when I prayed to Our Lady – and to Shaun – to take care of me, it was almost as though my smiling Shaun, as he was before, came out to help me. I had a definite feeling of Shaun looking after me.

Had a lovely evening last night. Pat and Julie took me to the Hengist for a lovely meal. Again, it was as though Shaun knew I was there. I know he would think they had given me such a treat – really as though they had kept his promise to me for him.

Matt and Jo are in Wales. Hope the weather holds.

Mike phoned from Australia this afternoon. Spoke to both him and Jill. Their son, Robert, has passed his driving test.

Sunday 7th

A thought: 50% of all married people have to endure the death of a spouse. In a way God has been so kind to me in the way we witnessed Shaun's passing. A miracle in itself. (I have really lost the thread of my thoughts here – I shall have to come back to this another time.)

Ann has just phoned from Milford. That is another thing. God has blessed me with Matt and Jo, now in Ireland. Ann reckons October '92 for a wedding!

Matt phoned from Rosslare.

Shaun's uncle Mallachy, and later Mallachy's daughter Joan, phoned from Ireland as Matt and Jo had visited them.

Dave and Mary came last night. A good evening, although Dave gets upset. Very emotional.

Monday 8th

Depths of despair today. Watching Egyptian video at school with the class – graves – and the awful thought of decomposing bodies. The body that had held me and hugged me and kept me close.

Stuart has German measles. More lost school time.

Tuesday 9th

You miss the hugs, kisses and conversational rapport. Maybe you could get that in another relationship which would, in effect, be a tribute to your marriage. What early days to think of this! It *does not mean* that I love Shaun any the less – in fact, I only wish he were here in body as well as in spirit. (I know he is here in spirit.) It is because his hugs and kisses, etc., meant so much to me that it is a big need within me.

Went to St Peter's Church, Bearsted, tonight for a bereavement meeting. I suppose I could contribute constructively.

Two Months to the Day

Friday 12th

You have to yield to God and let the passing over be so smooth and peaceful. Two months by the date. Am I strong enough? Funny how you still function.

Last night we went to Littlehampton and Brighton. A brilliant evening – looked at two schools, went to the local presbytery for a very nice meal, guided tour of the church with all its attendant history, and – a highlight – a late night visit to the beach followed by a drink in a pub with Fr Jim, Malcolm, Catherine and Tricia, and then brandy back here at midnight.

Monday 22nd

5.45 p.m.: I want to die. I want to be with Shaun. I cannot live without him. I am so miserable and feeling sorry for myself. Saw Michèal for the last time – he is off to Ireland before taking up his new position.

Leavers' concert at St Francis' School today.

Last night was Michèal's do – a church leaving social.

Saturday: Nick, Sue and Lizzie came and Matt and Jo are back from Ireland.

Friday night I was taken out by Ed and Sr Mary.

Tuesday 23rd

Life isn't fair. Why? Why must I do without my man to hold me? It is getting worse – a bad nightmare.

Last day of the school year. No way this time last year would my present status have entered my head. How can I cope? I want – or need – to be selfish (and I know what that means) but of course I can't.

Thursday 25th

Noreen brought the parasol to match the garden furniture tonight. She is a good friend and doesn't mind (I don't think) just talking and listening.

Have begun painting the hall.

Spoke to David Cunningham's secretary. Total money sent in Shaun's name was £1,745. She was really pleased.

Met Florrie yesterday and took her to the cemetery.

Out with Tony, Alice, Ian and Stuart tonight.

Sunday July 28th

A hard, but I suppose well-worthwhile weekend. Terry picked Stuart and me up on Friday night. Had two late nights at Guildford where they live and many tears with Terry.

Cranleigh today – nice to still keep in contact with Hank and Anne. I only hope they still feel the same and won't mind coming back to me even though Shaun won't be here. I wish with all my heart he was.

Had a letter from David Cunningham – he will never forget Shaun. **Nor will I!**

Life is hard – I need my man so much! How selfish can I get? Why can't I even share him?

Midnight: You are a widow. Get used to the word. No man in your bed to comfort you.

Tuesday 30th

6.00 p.m.: I have lost my husband, lover, best friend. Someone to moan at, moan with, share secrets with, who would pick me up – or put me down. To laugh with and to cry with, just to exist with and share his very being. I am now only half the person I was.

11.30 p.m.: Have been for a test drive in the new car with Chris – and have been out with Harry and Jean and their daughter Siobhan. I apologised for boring them with talk about Shaun – but they said it was good. He was human – not always good, thank goodness; he was just right, straight and level. I miss him and love him to death. I went to the cemetery and asked about a rose bush. £72.50 for ten years.

The sooner Matt and Jo get married, the more pleased I will be. They are already older than we were when we got married. Watched a replay of the 1966 World Cup Final today (25 years ago). Pity Shaun didn't see this. He always thought of '66 as his year. I hope to goodness Matt and Jo not only make their 25th but also their 40th. Thought we would have seen both. How wrong can you get?

What am I doing sitting here at 12.20 a.m. watching the '66 Cup Final if it isn't for you, my darling? I needed to do it for you.

12

Purgatory

Friday 2nd

The good thing is that if Shaun is a saint – and Michèal reckons he is – then thank God he is a *human* saint because at times he could be a sod. That must prove that God is caring – no human can be perfect from birth to death. What sort of a saint would that be? God knows the human potential – after all he created man in his own likeness. It gives me strength that people as caring and basically human as Shaun and Kathleen are now saints. I would like to take up this conversation with Fr Jim.

Mum and Dad have been down today. I took them to the cemetery and they took Stuart and me to the Running Horse. Had a good afternoon in the garden. We all tried hard.

Pick up new car tomorrow. I miss Shaun. No one to talk to, to bandy words with, lose my temper with, make love with. It is getting harder.

Out last night to Springfield Club with Noreen and Brenda. How can you write down all that you are missing? You have to go on because you are still here (haven't finished your purgatory). How do you explain the emptiness after living your life completely with someone for 24 plus years? Only half of you is left to carry on. How? Tonight, all of a sudden, I miss the physical side. How can I write this in my diary?? I need Shaun for his physical contact. After all these months I miss it. How do widows cope? I keep getting cheques – I'd rather have my man.

12.00 midnight. So tired – must go to bed.

Sunday 4th

Jo's parents, Ann and David, here this morning. Lovely to see them. Picked up the new car yesterday. Gradually getting used to it.

Monday 5th

Ordered stair carpet today. Think it will be ready before I've finished painting!

Went to see the dermatologist, Dr Conor O'Docherty of Dublin, today. He is off to Donegal tomorrow. Says I have a fungal infection – obviously made worse by smoking. No way did he lecture me – his brother-in-law died in the Marsden at the age of 44. Said they should have a monument to the patients who take the experimental treatment knowing deep down that they are doing it for others – no hope of a cure for them. A different perspective! He has prescribed fungilin tablets – Shaun would be laughing his head off. I used to nag him to take them – and then I'd find them after an hour in all sorts of strange places: beside the bed, down the loo, in the bin, ashtrays, etc.

He has got to be laughing – getting his own back! This has made me smile! I even enjoy this! I can share, in part, what he went through. Says that this fungus is not stress-related – pure coincidence – although I'm not sure.

10.45 p.m.: A big void. Dr O'Docherty was likening his sister-in-law's four young children to my teaching – both take your mind off things. Advised me to talk and talk (which I do), to write it all down (which I am doing), **and get on with living**. Hinting at finding another man perhaps? He says religion plays a big part and he is right.

Wednesday 7th

Last night Melanie and Kelly came. Both good girls – brought back good memories of Lourdes.

Ruby has been today. Very upset, worried about the future. Haven't done any more painting today although the carpet is ready. Getting cold feet about going to Wales. Don't want to go without Shaun – don't fancy the drive – and if I don't go Matt could get used to the car.

Thursday 8th

A lovely dream last night. Shaun was with me. It was very real, and it
wasn't the sick Shaun – it was my man as he was. Wish I could
remember all the details but I woke up happy. This is the second time
I have dreamt like this. I wish it could have been more often. I wonder
whether it is anything to do with praying to him? I asked him last
night to work out the right answer for Ruby and Frank. It was really
as if he was just around the corner waiting for me.

Went to 12.30 p.m. Mass today. It was said by Fr Brendan from
Aylesford and he said a special bidding prayer – said that the Mass
was being said for Shaun and that the whole parish were praying for
us as a family.

Teresa and the boys were there as well. Have rung Ann and told
her I am not coming to Wales. She understands that it's too soon for
me. She has bad toothache.

Saturday 10th

Tina and Peter brought their great friends June and Ray down this
morning. Roger, Caroline and Anthony came to dinner last night. A
good evening, they didn't leave until 1.50 a.m.

Fr Jim phoned in the afternoon. Thought I had sounded a bit down
earlier. We talked for ages – even about the diary on which this book
is based.

I went to the cemetery yesterday morning but I was too early at first
– they don't open until 10.00 a.m.

Well, the big cheque arrived today. A lot of money. But how can
you evaluate it with a life? It upsets me – it is as though this is what
Shaun was worth. Hard cash. What nonsense. I feel my emotions are
walking a very thin tightrope. I would just like to go to sleep and wake
up with my husband. Life is like a nightmare. I am even losing my
confidence about driving. How long will these feelings last? Will it
ever get any better? How do people cope? I really don't like being so
unhappy – not my old nature at all. Still haven't finished the decorating
– need the ladder now.

Sunday 11th

12.10 p.m.: I'm secretly pleased. Matt and Jo came back from Weymouth and Matt said he liked the new pictures I have put up in the hall. Someone else within the household to comment on things now that Shaun has gone. Three months today since my life changed beyond repair.

Went to borrow Teresa and Bryan's ladder this morning but Bryan did the last bit of painting for me.

Rose came to collect travelling plug and kettle. Stuart and I went to a pizza restaurant for lunch.

Geraldine phoned tonight – she's getting ready for Brittany. I spoke to Roger in Wales – he kept saying, 'you poor thing', when I told him why I wasn't going, but he completely understood. Delyth is not well again. Roger admits he gets irritable – I can understand only too well why. I feel for him. I wish they were nearer; I would love to give them a hug.

I've always lived and believed that you get what you earn. I haven't earned this money. I've got it – I don't want it – I want Shaun! Sod the money!

Monday 12th

Three calendar months. Still getting worse, not better yet. Stuart up very early to get early train to London to see Press Release of 'Terminator'. Paid the big cheque into the bank.

Went to Mass and spoke to Sister Eileen about Friday – our forthcoming trip to Aylesford Priory to see a performance of *The Mystery Plays* (re-enactment of Bible stories). Saw Fr Jim and he has asked me for lunch on Wednesday. I must try to be better company for him. He only sees my *down* side, which is a pity. I shouldn't really burden him, yet I can talk to him so honestly.

I am not even really straight in my own mind about what I want. If I were to wish away all the pain and heartache I am not sure that that would be right – not sure really that I want to – maybe it is a sort of self-punishment that I need to go through. Logically I know that that isn't right, yet . . . maybe it is a need I have to go through in order to come out the other side.

Matt drove the new car for the first time. Jo said he did alright. Something I wrote weeks and weeks ago in this diary – and I'm not sure why I wrote it then: 'the past has to give way to the future.' A basic statement – true in its core – yet is it not the past which makes us what we are in the future? I cannot give up the past, yet I must make a future for myself. A selfish statement when written baldly like that – yet I have to do it for others. What sort of a future? Certainly a different direction. A future without the man who made me what I am now – and I thank him for that at least. I know it is not his fault he has left me. I know there is a good reason unknown as yet to me. I will know one day. I wonder what the future holds? Please God help me to overcome all the problems. I know I have my own personal saint watching out for me. I talk to him all the time. That can't be wrong, can it? I wonder, is it right that I pray and talk to Shaun more for me than I pray for him? I seriously believe I do not need to pray for Shaun as much as for me because I *know* he is already in Heaven. I can't be doing with the morbid prayers. I really feel – and know – that he is with God and Our Lady. She is a great comfort to me. Our Lady of Lourdes has a great power of comfort.

Tuesday 13th

Went to buy Stuart's bike today and then the pair of us went to the Malta for lunch. Stuart was talking about his long-time friend Ian Baigent and how ages ago he said that when he was old enough he was looking forward to going for a drink with Shaun. Stuart's friends really did like Shaun. That was obvious on the school trip to the Isle of Wight a few years ago. There were a lot of Stuart's friends at the funeral. June and Dave, my aunt and uncle, called in this afternoon. Nice to see them. I managed to get all the old hall carpet up ready for tomorrow. Feelings don't get any less intense.

Wednesday 14th

New hall carpet fitted today. Had a lot of clearing up afterwards to do! Matt says he likes it.

Went to lunch with Fr Jim. Very pleasant – talked about everything and anything.

A thought: If Heaven is complete happiness, it follows that those who are there can feel no pain – not even the sadness of being apart from those they have loved here on Earth – so why are they waiting for us? Unless it is to welcome us into their blissful environment? What happens when someone marries again? Who does the welcoming? I suppose the all-encompassing love and happiness leave no room for jealousy.

I hope to goodness we are right in our beliefs of a life after death. Why am I asking this? We have proof – through the manner of Shaun's dying – of another, better life.

Thursday 15th

Went to London today with Stuart and we met Matt for lunch in The Old Shades in Whitehall. Nice. Visited Ruby briefly and she looks somewhat better.

Feast of the Assumption. I enjoyed Mass tonight; felt as though Shaun was with me. Although I really didn't like the first reading, I came out feeling quite uplifted.

Matt has said tonight that I have made a good job of the hall. Nice to be praised.

Saturday 17th

Last night – Aylesford Priory for *The Mysteries*. Very well done. Had a nice evening. Today, I've been depressed. Went to the cemetery, did a bit of gardening and not a lot else except sit under the tree and talk and think and cry. Sometimes I don't want to go on. I keep thinking of the future. Fatal really. No good thinking about our anniversary coming up – I should just take one day at a time.

Shaun's cousin Brian phoned tonight. Brian's brother Anthony has throat cancer. They thought at first it was a wart on his voice box but it was more serious than that.

Sunday 18th

Rock bottom.

Had a barbecue – first one without Shaun. First of the year as well. Maybe that is why I feel so bad. Cried my eyes out upstairs afterwards. Jo knew – she said it was early days.

I don't know what the point is to life except maybe as a kind of
Purgatory to get through – something better eventually.
Maybe I need help if I feel like this.

Monday 19th

I'm alive and living – in Britain, England, Kent, Maidstone. But why?
What purpose am I serving by being alive here? None that I can think
of.

Wednesday 21st

Yesterday Nick, Sue and Lizzie came. We walked to the Malta for
lunch. Nice.
  Phoned Delyth today; called into school. Matt and Jo staying at
Mum's tonight after a Simple Minds concert at Wembley. Met Sister
Eileen in town: do I want to go to Hythe with the Women's group in
October?
  Met Monica – she knows I am not right.
  Took Stuart to tennis and went to the cemetery in between dropping
off and picking up.
  Phoned David Cunningham's secretary after receiving last bill for
Shaun's treatment. Nice how BUPA point out that we have *almost*
used up the money – even though the letter was addressed to the
Executor of Shaun Ellesmere's Estate. Doesn't help how you feel. I
feel . . . nothing. I am no use to anyone at the moment – only when I
pretend.

Thursday 22nd

Am I the right person at the moment to be a teacher? I've been into
school a couple of times and spent two afternoons doing some work.
Teaching is alright for the few hours you are daily immersed in it and
then my other side has to surface, as wife and mother – but no longer
wife. Breadwinner, yes – but not wife. This is when I become a
different person.
  Both Elizabeth (Lionel's wife) and Julie phoned. Have told them
both that I am now beginning to realise that I will not see Shaun again

– he is not on a rugby trip. He has actually left me. How do I go on?
Why do I go on? For the boys. I miss out. I'm sure they do, too – but,
my God, I have such a big need.

Friday 23rd

Busy day. Went to Pauline's and Ron's for lunch – walked down the
Loose valley near Maidstone first for a drink and then back for lunch
and a haircut. Very pleasant.

Rosemary called in later and then cousin Ian and his wife Linda
arrived. Stuart and I went to the Running Horse for dinner. Fr Chris
was here when we arrived back.

Dave and Mary are coming tomorrow. Still getting BUPA bills and
tax forms.

Ian and Linda had been to the cemetery. They saw only one person
and two squirrels. They thought it was very peaceful.

Saturday 24th

A thought: once you make a decision to get married then your life
becomes a shared life. Everything is done bearing the other half in
mind – it cannot be any other way if it is a true commitment. What
happens, then, when you lose your partner? *Your* life is half gone and
really quite worthless.

Dave and Mary are coming later.

Tuesday 27th

2.00 p.m.: Had a lovely dream last night – made me wake up happy. I
had gone to collect Shaun from rugby, but it was a Blackheath pitch
and he hadn't been playing. Nigel and Terry, former Maidstone rugby
players, were in the dream. Shaun was dressed in bottle-green
trousers, not his cords, though, and we just sat around talking. I have
no recollection of what about, but we were all well and in good, happy
moods. It would be nice if I could dream of Shaun more often, but
you can't make them to order.

Matt is off at the moment taking his driving test. Hope he succeeds.

He and Jo came back from Wales last night – they had been to Jo's brother Steve's 21st.

Met the new priest on Saturday. He is from Erith and plays rugby for Bexley.

Mary, a friend from church, phoned Sunday. I must try to go out with her – I'm sure she could give me some advice.

Mary is back in hospital. She now has cancer in the fluid around the spinal cord. What a destructive disease! How long before it can be eradicated I wonder?

Thursday 29th

Have had a nice day. Julie and her youngest son Patrick arrived and we went to the Malta for lunch. As we were walking back we were talking and I said that I thought that by now people who visited or phoned me would be wearing off, but they aren't and she said it was because I was good company – people did not do things out of a sense of duty. Nice thought.

Suzanne, a friend from school days, came yesterday and so did Nick, Sue and Lizzie. Nick brought the next instalment of this diary, which he has been printing out for me.

Had a good evening Tuesday when Ed and Sister Mary came to dinner. I have felt better this week than last – probably because it is almost time to go back to school.

Friday 30th

5.40 p.m.: Why did God need *you*? He didn't need me! I have to stay here! Yet, I wouldn't want you to go through the pain I go through now – so if it had to be one of us, I suppose I am (grudgingly) glad that you were chosen instead of me. Serves me right for saying I felt better yesterday – today I don't.

Have sent a letter to David Cunningham wondering why four people in our avenue have died of liver cancer within a year if it is so rare?

Spoke to Jill from down the road today. She feels she is ready to move now – over three years since her husband died. She dreams of pulling her husband back and he is saying he can't but he is alright – she must make a new life for herself.

Saw Fr Chris today. Another Mass for Shaun will be on Friday – Fr Michèal's offering.

I have booked a Mass for October 29th and also one as a Christmas present for Shaun on the weekend before we fly to Australia.

Saturday 31st

A bad, bad day all day; it is funny but I don't know why some days are like this. It has been bad (in a sad way) really since I got up. Tears just spring to my eyes with no real reason. Later, Noreen phoned with a message that Mary wanted to talk to me. I phoned her and spoke to both her and Steve. She was saying that in June the Marsden were thrilled that the type of cancer she had in the lungs and the bones was in remission and that this was very unusual. But then, five weeks ago, cancer cells in small clusters were found in the fluid in the spinal column. (She had gone back to the hospital after having tingling sensations in her feet. Hearing this reminded me of Shaun saying that he often felt as though the soles of his feet were flapping.) The hospital said it was nothing to worry about but a fortnight ago they found it had spread through the fluid into the brain.

Mary is now on a harsh course of radiotherapy and is staying in the Marsden during the week and coming home at weekends. She sounded okay on the phone and is determined to fight on. She was talking about quality of life but said also that the doctors can't do it on their own – she has to do her part. Mary says she is doing it for Shaun. My God, I wish her so well – but I feel so helpless. I don't know if I can believe any more that cancer can be truly beaten. I have felt awkward about talking to her and Steve because I feel I must be a bad reminder of what can happen to them but she said she wanted to talk to me and to see me. I have promised I will phone next week.

Josephine was here this afternoon. I do so enjoy being with her – she understands. I said I must stop feeling so sorry for myself but she said, 'Why should you? I certainly would!'

I miss him so much. Apparently Mary has said 'The dying is easy; it is the living that is hard.' That is so true also of those left behind. The living is torture at times.

13

Still Early Days?

Tuesday 3rd

Things like paying bills, paper work, etc., I can cope with because I always did. So I have that to be grateful for – not something I have suddenly had to take on board and learn. However, things that affect the boys, Shaun always helped me with. If they had something wrong with them I, as a mum, worried overmuch; he had the calming, stable instinct of a male who puts things into a logical perspective. Consequently, Stuart has had X-rays on his knees today and I worry. Shaun would have reassured me.

Had RE day today at the neighbouring Catholic school, Holy Family, with Sr Maura, religious education coordinator for the diocese. She asked how Shaun was – she hadn't heard.

Wednesday 4th

First day with new class. They are young!!

Had a lovely letter from Mary today. She is so positive and fighting because Shaun was so full of life and she wants to continue for him. Spoke to Steve tonight. He has been for another job interview.

Vicky phoned – worried about what will happen to her when the firm is taken over. Mum and Dad have finished their decorating.

Thursday 5th

Spent over an hour at the solicitors. I still have over £9,800 to pay on the mortgage! Didn't apparently have protection, on the loans for house extension, improvements, etc. Lloyds' stuff still not sorted out either (documentation relating to Shaun's once having been a 'name').

Went to cemetery – the headstone is beautiful. I am really pleased.

Fr Jim phoned – needed to talk to me for a few minutes. Mìcheal has given up the priesthood and wanted us to know before gossip reached us; he said I had done a lot for him. I hope people support him in his decision – not something he would have taken lightly. 'A reluctant priest' as Shaun called him, but maybe because of that a stronger one. I hope all goes well for him. Nice of Fr Jim to come. Spoke to him briefly about the Catholic Truth Society's Widow's pamphlet.

Saturday 7th

Went to see Mary today. She was not well – but exuded a peaceful feeling. Steve had his outward face on.

Went to cemetery this morning to put flowers in front of the headstone. Someone (it has to be Vicky) has put a cut-glass vase there already.

Lionel and Elizabeth came to dinner last night. The firm has been taken over – all jobs are safe for the moment.

Mrs D. is having an operation on her cheekbone after slipping over in the hospital.

Sunday 8th

2.30 p.m.: I've lived through so much since the Lourdes photo was taken. I wish I was back there – as things were – but with a different outcome. I am so full of self-pity – I know Shaun is alright but I need him!

I dislike Sundays. I can't help thinking of the old Sundays; Shaun spending the morning in the garden while I pottered in the kitchen; he coming in at about 1.00 p.m. for his pint and a phone call to his Mum, and then – a big dinner and we'd settle down for the afternoon for a quiet, cuddled time. Now this will never happen again. I am so lonely. Sunday was, I suppose, our day of togetherness – although if

I'm honest, there were a lot of Sundays I didn't enjoy. Maybe I need the routine of a working life. I know I need my man. You do miss the physical side. That is an admission of a personal nature, but it can't just be written off. I need Shaun's physical contact – and I say Shaun's because that is the only contact I've had. How can I go on? Think of it as Purgatory? Serving it now must mean you don't have it still to come – surely?

Tuesday 10th

Mum, Dad, Tina and Peter called in yesterday after their trip to Beltring. They had been to the grave and liked the headstone. Tonight Teresa and I have been to Fr Chris for another bereavement meeting. I feel these meetings need to be structured from now on.

One thing that a woman said when talking about her brother-in-law and the funny colour of his feet reminded me of the nurse on the Saturday afternoon, May 11th, saying that it wouldn't be long before Shaun died because of the look of his legs – quite purple really. Pat said the nurse told her it was a sign of the body shutting down. Not a bad way of putting it.

11.55 p.m. Trouble is, *being so practical*, I need to know how long I have to endure – carry on – without my man? Death has to be the easy way out.

Friday 13th

Isn't it strange, how you can be surrounded by people, be very busy, have lots of visitors and phone calls – and yet still be terribly, utterly lonely?

Had a good evening on Wednesday with Tony, Alice and her brother Gerrard. Went to The Wheelers.

Saw Dr Gardner yesterday for the results of Stuart's X-rays. They seem clear but blood samples have been taken to test for arthritis.

Sue's birthday. Sent flowers.

Feel down today.

Spoke to Steve yesterday. He has been very down – I know exactly how he feels.

Sunday 15th

3.30 p.m.: Death gives another dimension to life. We spend life in a rush – no time to stop and care, stop and think, stop and talk. I regret that now – I will take time to do these things. What a hard lesson to learn.

I wasn't well yesterday – gastric flu I think. Bit better today. Pat gave us good news after church tonight. Michèal is starting work for him tomorrow – selling stone!

Roger and Delyth are coming for a few days before half term. Will be good to see them.

Wednesday 18th

My poor darling; he wasn't ready to die. Correction. In the last 10 days he was. Quote from a play I'm watching about the disabled visiting the shrine at Knock: 'Not God or fate, but bloody bad luck.' Very true. Had a wonderful surprise on Monday. Michèal arrived as I was cooking dinner; very nervous but he soon relaxed. We opened the champagne – had had no reason to do so before. He had spent his first working day and had enjoyed it. Gave me lots of hugs – knew it was what I needed. I took him up to see Teresa.

Have had meetings after school every night. Fr Jim has been good again. Had a nice card from Sue – 'Thinking of you'.

Sunday 22nd

A thought: Shaun had a certain amount of intolerance – but only because he had certain values and would not believe in compromising them. A very straight person.

Shelagh came on Friday. We went to the cemetery and then to Waldorfs for a meal. A nice evening. Josephine called in Saturday afternoon with a present of an amber necklace from Poland – 1,200 years old.

Last night Fr Jim came to dinner. It was a lovely evening – very good conversation. He is very good company.

An Unhappy Anniversary

Monday 23rd

5.20 p.m.: Okay, the date is one day out but it was on this correspond-
ing Monday last year that Dr Powell-Jackson told us of definite secondary cancer of the liver and that there was nothing that could be done.
A year ago? What a lot I've been through since. Why? Don't know –
must remember the prayer (which is printed on Shaun's headstone):

Then Shall I Know

Not till the loom is silent
And the shuttles cease to fly,
Shall God unroll the canvas
And explain the reason why.
The dark threads are as needful
In the weaver's skilful hands
As the threads of gold and silver
In the pattern he has planned.

I hate feeling so lonely, miserable and depressed. I was saying to Fr
Jim on Saturday that really I was lucky – in the manner of Shaun's
going – but I don't feel lucky now. Just empty. Where do all the tears
come from?

Tuesday 24th

10.50 p.m.: Breda, Mary's great friend, has been. I had phoned Steve
last night and got the answerphone – yet I had guessed he was there.
Mary has been given just weeks but she doesn't know yet. Steve didn't
know how to tell me, thought it would bring back memories. That is
wrong – the memories are constant – I would rather help. I would
rather be needed, but at the same time I don't want to interfere. I have
written to him anyway. How will he cope with the loneliness? He will
be alright for a few months – but after that?

Sue and Nick have had their garage broken into and Nick's bike has
been stolen – rough justice after Sunday, when he helped me get a
new bike for Stuart.

Wednesday 26th

Steve phoned last night; it took courage, I think, for him to talk to me. I feel for and identify so much with him. It gets worse: I thought Shaun was far too young at 47 to lose his life, but Mary is only 34. And yet the Government is talking about having to make provision for so many more people living over the age of 70. We must just be the unlucky ones – especially if we live to be that age!

Dave phoned tonight. He has got promotion – Assistant Chief Constable in Newcastle. I wish him well. He moves in three weeks.

Saw Dr Gardner tonight. Stuart's blood tests are all clear. Spoke to my solicitor. Looks as though I had better pay off the mortgage – almost £10,000. All I'll get in return is about £1,700 mortgage protection. Not what either Shaun or I ever expected. We thought we were covered.

Saturday 28th

Not a very good day. Very wet so I don't suppose that helps. New washing machine/dryer fitted. Boys and Jo have gone to watch Spurs. I went to the cemetery. The plot next to Shaun is now occupied – the grandmother of a little girl in school. I felt quite upset up there today. Re-read Shaun's letter to old school friend Micky in Australia. Incredible to think he wrote it only a few weeks before he died – yet he still thought he had odds of 2–1 and was talking about having his 50th birthday and how soon after that he could retire.

9.45 p.m.: Brian has just phoned. He asked what I was thinking about. I told him I had a touch of melancholia – watching people in a film on the television enjoying New Year's Eve. Anthony has had 15 of 23 treatments. His voice should come back. Brian has an interview on Monday with Tate and Lyle – to drive the managing director.

Back to the melancholia. Brian said I would have to enjoy the New Year, etc. Okay. The shell of me will. I can put on a show. Inside will be empty. Like a dried up nut. Looks good on the outside – until you use the nutcrackers.

Have just spoken to Steve. Mary hasn't been too bad today; he is pretending, but he enjoyed a day's work yesterday. I know exactly how he feels. What can I do? History repeating itself.

12.15 p.m.: Actually I now feel rotten. I've just looked at Shaun's photo and sworn at him! He looked so alive that the fact he has died is so unreal! He should still be here – then I could nag him normally! I love him so much.

Sunday 29th

Hank and Anne came for coffee on their way to Walderslade near Chatham. They had been to the cemetery and were both tearful. I was already feeling the same way. I wonder why some days are worse than others? I suppose I have more time to just think at the weekend. Jo's Mum, Ann, phoned at lunch time. Speaking to Jo about weddings. Good job Matt was at football practice! Jo has developed a bad cold tonight.

My turn to read at Mass tonight. Showed Fr John the nice letter I had from Pat C. of Bexley Rugby Club. I will write to him.

Monday 30th

Noreen had been north to see her brother. They left at 7.30 a.m. in the morning but he died at 8.00 a.m. What rotten news. Teacher Pauline Holliday in on supply today. She is nice to talk to – very understanding.

Keep thinking of Steve. Dreamt that Michèal phoned last night. It seemed very real. I would like to talk to him but he has a different life to lead now.

11.30 p.m.: Funny, I get really tired after a day at school and I look forward to reading in bed, but I keep putting off the time I go. Is it loneliness which keeps me away from by bed? Probably. And the warmth. And the comforting cuddles. Emptiness.

14

Shaun would have Enjoyed the Rugby

Tuesday 1st

5.30 p.m.: I know why I've been upset today. Des phoned at lunchtime offering the three of us tickets for the World Cup Rugby match – England v Italy – at Twickenham.

I had a few tears on the coach coming back from the school field. Malcolm noticed. It was because I was thinking how much Shaun would have loved to see the matches in this Cup. Also I remember him saying to me, 'Tell Malcolm I owe him a pint', when he was good to me one morning when I was upset.

Wednesday 2nd

6.00 p.m.: Cancer might take our bodies but it will *never* get our souls. That is one way the despicable disease is definitely beaten.

More letters via the solicitor again today. One to sign for £1,700 insurance – all that is left of mortgage protection; and one to sign for Lloyds name business. Probably be just my luck that I have to pay out the £17,000+ on that! Have sent off a cheque for nearly £10,000 today to clear the mortgage.

Saw Fr Jim early this morning, while getting a Mass card for Noreen. Has asked if I would – if it wouldn't offend my sensibilities – read a document about the new Hospice in Maidstone and give my comments. I've said I would.

11.00 p.m.: Pauline has been to give me a perm and cut Stuart and Jo's hair.

Steve phoned. He and Mary's mother have been bullying her to get up and dressed and she has eaten well today. I am going over tomorrow evening. Sr Kathleen has been to see her this evening and told Steve that I had had a *down* day yesterday, so he was phoning to cheer me up.

Spoke to Sine about the rugby tickets her husband Des had provided. Thanked her.

Thursday 3rd

Went to see Mary and Steve tonight. A nice enjoyable hour plus Mary looked a lot better than I had expected. She has been eating – had one piece of the chocolate I took for the boys and was drinking her first cup of tea for over four weeks. I think Steve still has a few more weeks with her yet. Steve looked shattered – yet ready for a laugh. It is this false world we live in; the outward face is on show – inwardly you're shrivelling up. He could joke about the nurses making him miss the first six points scored today by England against New Zealand in the opening match but I know he would have willingly given up that rugby if only his life could run smoothly.

I hope I'm right over him still having a few weeks yet. I can only base it on my own experience with Shaun. If Mary follows the same pattern then that statement is true. However, I don't know – as Mary now has cancer in the brain – whether the pattern is set to follow the same path. In a way, I hope it is, because the dying was peaceful, dignified and almost right in a strange way. No horrific scenes to witness. I still don't know how we would have coped if things had been different.

Fr Jim gave me the philosophy of the new Maidstone Hospice to comment on. I have done it, but I don't think it will do him any good.

Fr John tells me he saw Shaun's photo in Bexley club last night.

11.40 p.m.: Sitting here watching a recording of England versus All Blacks with tears in my eyes. Shaun wanted to see this so much. My man – has he really missed it? Or is he actually watching it from his nice, comforting position away from this man-led fallible world?

Friday 4th

6.00 p.m.: I was woken up from a lovely dream this morning. So real. Shaun was with me; I was woken up too early for a successful conclusion. These dreams – so few and far between – are so real. A reminder of life as it really was – and cannot be again.

St Francis' Feast Day. Whole school – Fr John's first school Mass and he did very well. Steve was there. I felt low, listening to the children's versions of the prayer to St Francis.

Terry was on the phone tonight about the Ireland trip. He will call in with Florrie tomorrow.

12.00 p.m.: **midnight**: Shelagh and Pete have just left – nice evening in Waldorfs but I have not been good company. It can't be the same for them – coming without Shaun being here. It isn't the same for me either; no husband to turn to. Especially after this morning's dream – which didn't reach fruition – I really am lonely. What can I do?

Went to see Fr Jim after school with my report on the new Hospice. He is happy with the current architects of the new church.

Sunday 6th

Yesterday was eventful. I went to the cemetery first. It was raining but I changed the flowers. After I'd done the week's ironing I went to see Mary. She is keeping up appearances but she is weak. Her legs have got so thin.

Terry and Florrie arrived and then Steve brought his Mum, Kath, over to see them.

Fr John came to supper. Played Stuart on the computer.

Today, Steve, Jo's brother, came to dinner and to watch Wales lose rugby to Western Samoa. Ireland won their match.

Peter H. is in the Marsden. Not good news apparently.

When I read these words back they seem so clinical – just factual sentences. They're a true account of what really did happen, but they take no account of feelings.

I wonder if I'll ever be happy again? I suppose so, but it is hard to see how. I really get tearful on Sunday mornings – memories of hugs at the kitchen sink and then watching Shaun through the window as he gardened and I cooked the Sunday dinner. A real sadness comes over me. Such an emptiness in my life, and it can never be filled again by Shaun.

Monday 7th

5.00 p.m.: I must have woken up three or four times last night with cold feet! Is there no end to the reasons for which I miss Shaun? I suppose if I can come through the 29th – our 25th anniversary – then I might be on the way up.

Have just realised that it is a year ago today that we had that early morning drive to the Marsden. First time I met Steve and Mary.

Spoke to Ed and Sr Mary at Parent-Teacher Association AGM at St Simon Stock School.

Spoke to Steve. He told me not to get maudlin.

Tuesday 8th

I own, I suppose, a house and a car. The only reason I own them is because I have a husband no more. Guess what I'd rather have?

The school Mass this morning was for Shaun, but at communion Fr John made a big thing about it and asked the children to pray for us. I got upset – natural I suppose because I miss him so much. Went to the archives and ordered Mike's photocopies today.

The boys and Jo went to Twickenham to see England beat Italy. They met my brother Nick and Mick Brett (an old school friend of mine and Shaun's) on the way. Hearing about friends like Mick always reminds me that Shaun and I went to the same primary school. Steve was taking Mary to the Marsden today. That shows a good deal of courage on her part.

Roger phoned – Delyth's father has died. The supply work is going to stop in Wales. Delyth is studying for a degree in French and Business Studies!

More Sad News amid Daily Life

Wednesday 9th

'Come back and stay for *good* this time': a Paul Young record being advertised on TV at the moment. Funny how you can twist the words. I know it isn't possible, but how I wish it were. 'You learn a lot from the dying.' A quote from Noreen tonight on the phone. And something I believe.

Tony S. phoned – still talking about the funeral and the measure of the man – to let me know that Simon, his son, is now at East Anglia University studying economics.

Then, out of the blue, Tamsin phoned, asking me to be her sponsor at her confirmation on Sunday. I was honoured and overwhelmed to be asked. I told her she had caused tears of happiness. I first rang Noreen, who thought it would be a good idea, and she knew I was upset – in a nice way. Consequently she later turned up here. A good friend indeed.

I phoned Sr Mary to let her know. She now hopes to be at the confirmation. She spoke about Peter Hanna, the other man on the Lourdes trip suffering from cancer. It has now gone to his throat. He cannot speak and his wife now has had a cancerous growth removed. Two children, one has just left school and the other one is in the second year of St Simon Stock.

Noreen brought two story books over from Fr Chris for me to read with regard to Mary's boys. (The books are specially written for children on the subject of bereavement.) They have come from the Macmillan nurses. One would be okay – one needs to be reworded. I'll see him tomorrow.

11.20 p.m.: Time to go to bed – and dream. Of what? An empty future.

Friday 11th

5.30 p.m.: Funny, Fridays used to be a time of relaxing in the evening. All the family safely gathered in; time to sit and unwind after a week's work. Now, I'm looking for company – something to do – even though I'm still just as tired after a busy week. Tomorrow, by the date, will be five months. Is it only 20 short weeks? 20 weeks is such a short period of time, yet I feel so drained, so useless – half a person without Shaun. And yet if this is only 20 weeks I have to think it could well be 20 years or more before being reunited. How do you cope with that thought?

Last night I went to Fr Chris at Bearsted – good. Quite a structured evening (bereavement meeting).

Terry B. phoned – talked about a hypodermic syringe being found on his school site and a teacher pricking herself. She now has to have months of Aids tests. I phoned Steve. He seems alright. I have phoned Pat G. to see if any temporary work would be available for him.

Simon was off school. He has had his leg set in plaster after a football accident on his knee.

England are through to the quarter-finals of the Rugby World Cup. Shaun would have loved it.

Sunday 13th

Tamsin's confirmation. Bittersweet feelings – Lourdes in the front of my mind. Who would have believed that five weeks after Lourdes Shaun was to die? Tamsin looked well – quite bubbly. She is a lovely girl. Spoke to Archbishop Bowen for a while.

Steve and Mary actually made it. Her eyes show the true extent of her illness. Yesterday I went to see them. She was determined to turn up today. I had quite a talk with Steve – life is hard for him. I'm not sure he has a steadfast faith. Who can blame him really? I suppose that is where I am lucky. Lucky! What an empty word. Deep down I know bloody well I'm not lucky. It's the question of two faces again – the pretend one is almost always on show.

Had a good evening last night. Trivial Pursuits at St Simon Stock. Our team didn't do very well, but we enjoyed the wine. Went back to the L.'s and didn't get home until almost 1.00 a.m.
11.30 p.m.: 'Decisions, decisions' – Shaun's famous saying. Not understanding, not wanting to make it – and yet he had that final strength from somewhere to make the big one, *at the right time for himself.*

Monday 14th

Brian phoned last night. Anthony has lost his job due to his son crashing his firm's car.

Mass at lunchtime for Shaun. Ruby was there and I met her after school for a coffee. Things haven't really changed for her. Have just spoken to Ann again. She is to have a week off at least. I told her she has to put herself and the baby first.

I suppose I'm a bit Jekyll and Hyde-ish! At work I think that for 99% of the time I function as I always did. Do they realise how I feel or react or behave when I come home? I wonder. I have not got my man to come home to.
11.40 p.m.: Funny how God can deal you such a blow yet *you still believe inherently.*

Tuesday 15th

John L. came today and has mended all my leaks. He is a very nice person. Went to the archives and got all the photocopying done for my brother Mike's proposed history book.

Little Laura was upset in Mass today. I spoke to her afterwards – she knows her Grandmother is buried next to Shaun and that they are in Heaven. I told her that any time she was fed up to come and talk to me – and if I was fed up I would talk to her. She smiled and cheered up. I hope that was the right way to tackle it.

Spoke to Jim and Wendy T. tonight. Apparently Jim was down a few weeks ago, had called in but I must have been at school. Spoke to Steve. Mary is okay. He said Michèal had been yesterday morning. I'm glad he did that, even though I haven't seen him again.

Letter from Melanie. Am going to write to her now.

11.40 p.m. At one stage you think – why did I fall in love with this particular person? Someone who was going to die early? If I had chosen someone else then I would still have a husband and my children would still have a father. Yet, my having chosen Shaun, who God in turn chose to take early, must mean that God wanted and needed him at this stage and therefore I had chosen right – I had chosen a man whom God had also chosen. Does that make sense? It does to me.

Wednesday 16th

11.15 p.m.: Have had a nice evening out with Paul and Brenda E. We went to the Golden Eagle at Burham. Have been there once before with Shaun – Malaysian food. Very good. They are good company, but it was their treat. I feel that people are spoiling me even though they say they are enjoying it. I feel beholden. I said I feel at times like a spare part, yet that is too strong – Paul and Brenda and other friends don't make me feel that way. Rather it is something within me that does it. In fact people go overboard to include me – I'm the one at fault.

Mary and Dave are coming for dinner on Friday.

It is now 11.45 p.m. I am sitting here, not really concentrating on anything on the television. I know I should go to bed as I am tired, but what is the point? Bed is lonely; Shaun is not there. I wish I could have the nice dreams about him more often.

Friday 18th

Come back to me please! It is so lonely, even with such good people around.

10.55 p.m.: Had a good time with Dave and Mary. I don't suppose I'll see them for a while. Dave goes to Northumbria on Sunday. Spoke to one of our former priests, Fr Peter S., briefly yesterday.

Mary will miss Dave before she joins him in Newcastle but she knows that at least she will see him again! I wish I could see and hold Shaun again now. I'm feeling sorry for myself again now!

Terry and Geraldine are going away to Scotland in the morning.

Saturday 19th

A bitterly cold wind at the cemetery this morning. Teresa and Peter were there as well. All the flowers were still fresh. I had to force the new ones in.

Saw Steve and Mary. Mary says she is not worried about the boys – there are plenty of people to love and care for them. With one breath she spoke about eating and exercising to get her strength up and the next she says she doesn't want to be here. It wouldn't surprise me if she has only a few weeks. Steve said he thought she'd had a stroke on Wednesday. The doctor said to expect more attacks.

Time to Change the Routine?

Sunday 20th

11.00 p.m.: What to write? Another Sunday. I sometimes wonder if I can get through them. It seems to be the worst day of the week. I always feel at my lowest. I wonder if I'm going round the bend? Everything seems so pointless on a Sunday. I'll have to think about changing the routine. Actually the fact that I've always been one for routine is something which probably makes things worse for me. If only I could have had more of a devil-may-care outlook – doing things more on the spur of the moment! Then I might not be having these feelings now about Sundays. I know Shaun used to nag me about being so routine-orientated. He has been proved right.

Julie phoned this evening. Pat and Mick B. have tried desperately hard to get Cup Final tickets. I really am grateful to them.

Wednesday 23rd

11.40 p.m.: Haven't had a chance to write for a few days. Roger and Delyth arrived on Monday. Lovely to see them, although they found it strange being here – they kept expecting to see Shaun. We went to the Bull last night – but we talked when we came back. I couldn't help getting upset. I still feel like a spare part without him although it's nobody's fault. Half of me has gone. They are safely home now. I like them a lot.

Had School Governors' meeting tonight. Fr Jim had to leave to go to the hospital – a mother in labour whose baby would either be born dead or die within a few hours. Got home to find Fr John here. He had been training at Bexley Rugby Club and had brought back the photo of Shaun and a lovely letter from Pat C. The photo must have been taken in the spring of '66 – 25 years before Shaun died – just a few months before we married. Nostalgia tinged with great sadness. Oh God, why me?

Thursday 24th

5.50 p.m.: Looking at the leaves on the trees and bushes dying down. I can see the wonder of nature – knowing that in springtime they will flourish again. I was going to say that it is a pity nature does not do the same for man. But, I suppose it does: through your children you live on – a new generation flourishes.

11.00 p.m.: Spoke to Steve. He couldn't speak freely but he sounded down. Things are obviously not right. Is it nearly time for Mary? He didn't really know.

Friday 25th

5.20 p.m.: Have had a lot of running around today because Florrie's phone has been cut off. It does not seem that she has paid the bill, however, so I will have phone calls to make and letters to write. Anyway, she has been reconnected now.

I feel so tired – end of the first half term. It has gone quickly – only tired, though, because the week stretched ahead. Matt and Jo are off to Wales tonight. Terry is 50 today. We should be thankful he has made it. Have had a lovely pair of silver earrings from Tina and Peter. I know why silver – although she was careful enough not to mention it.

Saturday 26th

11.00 p.m.: Didn't wake up until gone 9.00 a.m. Usual day – went to cemetery. Was thinking a lot today about last year in Stratford-on-Avon, although rethinking it at this time of night reminds me of the Hickman line and the time Shaun first forgot to clamp! The early hours of the morning in Stratford. My poor man – we didn't realise then what a short time we had left.

Went to the T.'s. Steve's brother was there as well as his Mum and Dad. Stupid, but I envied them a happy family life. Mary had just got up but she couldn't cope with visitors – so quiet and not with it. I really don't think she has very long.

Matt phoned from Wales. Jo's Mum and Dad have told him about his birthday present (tickets for the World Cup Rugby final) and he sounded over the moon!

Josephine brought me flowers for my anniversary next Tuesday. Daniel is staying tonight. Mass for Shaun. Fr Chris is back from America. He said the Mass.

Sunday 27th

Nick, Sue and Lizzie down this morning. They brought a rose bush – 'Whiskey Galore' – and a silver photo frame. We shed a few tears. Took Daniel (Josephine's son) and Stuart to a pizza restaurant for lunch.

Have been looking through the photos tonight to find one for the frame. That caused a few tears as well but I found a nice one taken in Stratford a year ago. What little time we really had, without even knowing it would end as it did. Life is unfair.

Monday 28th

Bought myself a gold locket in anticipation of tomorrow. After all, I won't get a gold anniversary. Did some more painting in the kitchen. Matt and Jo are getting engaged tomorrow! We are going for a meal. It has lifted my spirits really. Matt asked Jo's father David at the weekend. The wedding will be either next October or the following April. Something to look forward to. Spending next summer holidays making a wedding dress! What lovely news.

Wendy has spent the evening with me. She has driven down from Scotland to see her daughters in Kent. She is good company and knows exactly how I feel. She was doing bereavement counselling at one point and spoke of a lady who felt as though part of her had gone with her husband. Rather like my 'empty nut' theory. But Wendy asked her to think if that was really what her husband would have wanted. And of course it is not. As Wendy said, 'when I told her that you had told Shaun it was alright that he could go, she said that that was what she had got to tell herself'. In a way, I have to let go – not forget, but let go of *what has been* and move forward. Shaun will let me know when it is time for that; it is too soon at the moment, but, funnily enough, I had already had a 'chat' to him earlier today asking him where I go from here. When it is time he will let me know. I know he wouldn't want me to be an empty shell for ever. Somehow, the old me, and all it stood for, warts and all, has got to come back.

Spoke to Steve earlier. Mary is tired but they have been Christmas shopping. Says he is thinking of me with regard to tomorrow.

12.35 a.m.: Shaun has answered me very quickly. Considering I only asked/prayed to him at 5.00 p.m.: I now *know* that he would not want me to dwell in the past. I think he has 'spoken' doubly tonight – through both Matt and Jo and through Wendy.

Friends Make a Sad Day Less Painful

Tuesday 29th

Sue phoned early – 8.15 a.m. – and I gave her the good news about Matt and Jo. She shed a few tears. Fr Jim phoned just after 9.00 a.m. to see how I was. In fact the day was 50% better than I could ever have dreamt possible. Went to Mass. Fr John, Teresa, Sr Eileen and Sr Kathleen made everything worthwhile. Took three red roses to the cemetery. Terry arrived unexpectedly armed with flowers. He came with us to The Walnut Tree at Yalding for a meal – but he paid before he disappeared home. That was not the intention at all.

It is now 11.30 p.m. I don't know really how I feel. I **know** today is better than I could have envisaged but I **know** Shaun has helped me through it and I **know** I miss him terribly. Spoke to Steve earlier. He has funerals to attend.

Wednesday 30th

What's to say? I went to London today. Met Janet for lunch. Okay – until we said our goodbyes. Just after I got in, Steve arrived straight from a cremation. We talked – about work, the children, funerals and how life is for him at the moment. Trying to tear the walls down. I think I know – I've been there. Life is the killer. A paradox in words, but truth none the less.

Thursday 31st

12.05 a.m.: Everything can be ticking along fairly smoothly and all of a sudden a great wave of emotion hits you without any warning – I miss my man.

Mary and Julie took me to lunch today. They came bearing presents galore. Went to Mass tonight for the Eve of All Saints. Fr Chris said the Mass and I read the second reading.

Thinking of Steve. He will have all this still to go through. Is there a natural progression – a gradual easing? I suppose that on the surface there is – the outward face – how you appear (funny if someone says, 'it's nice to hear you sounding happy', you instantly feel guilty). Inwardly it is still so hard – no cuddles or hugs or reassuring words.

15
How can I Help Others who are Suffering?

Friday 1st

Mum, Dad, Pam and Bob were down today. We went to The Running Horse for lunch. They brought lots of presents.

Mick B. rang tonight. Had a long talk. He is a very good conversationalist. He will try to meet up with Matt and Jo tomorrow.

It is hard to describe how I feel. I am carrying on, yet why? What for? Living is empty. I think I have become very good at pretending while others are around. Yet inwardly I need Shaun – the closeness to another human being is something very hard to do without.

11.15 p.m.: The Rugby World Cup final has just been billed as the most important sporting event since the Football World Cup in 1966. That was a good year. Not like this.

I suppose that, much as I think that living on earth is Purgatory, if you aren't born and don't get the chance to *know* that, then what is it all really about? Does that make sense? Without having to live – or even being born to this earthly life – then I suppose you would never reach the ultimate goal of Heaven? Or would you? Surely not – if you've never been born then surely Heaven would be non-existent?

Saturday 2nd

I feel I let myself down today. I went to see Mary and Steve after going to the cemetery. Mary seemed much better than last week. She asked

me to stay and watch the Rugby Cup final, but I couldn't – and not
because England lost. I didn't know how I would react. I cried in front
of them which was very unfair of me. I shouldn't do that to them.

Tuesday 5th

11.15 p.m.: Have just had a long chat with Fr Jim. I had rung him
earlier, ostensibly to talk about the Hospice (which had been on television) and the positive outlook the patients had. He spoke a lot about
Shaun again and the manner of his dying. I think Shaun left a great
impression on him. I really should – when I can – ask Fr Jim a question:
how does God expect me to cope without him? It is a question of me
being able to drop the mask and be totally honest. Actually, maybe
bereavement turns you into a bit of a liar: you don't really want people
to suffer as much as you do, so you pretend – you talk about everyday
matters. You get on with life, you say you are okay, you do not drop
the facade – but inside you let go, *and can admit only to yourself* exactly
how devastated your life has become.

Yesterday I saw Dr O'Docherty again – he says he doesn't think I
have a pre-cancerous condition. He mentioned blood tests but then
said I didn't need them.

Wednesday 6th

Enjoyed our pilot scheme on swapping classes today. Phoned Steve
tonight. He has had the doctor out twice today to Mary – she hasn't
been out of bed and is now being sick.

Vicky and Dick from Shaun's firm were here tonight. Dick was
relating his happy memories of Shaun. There is uncertainty within
the firm. It will no longer carry the name 'Leadenhall' after January.
Dick said things have definitely changed.

Had a letter from school friend Betty W. – St Ursula's, 1956–1961 –
with a whole list of classmates and details of many marriages, jobs,
births, etc. Why, out of all those names, am I the only one whose
husband has died. Unfair, such loneliness.

Thursday 7th

Even now I can't always believe I will never see Shaun again. At school, Mr D. took an assembly to give us a bit of free time. I was talking to Noreen and broke down – the strains of the hymn wafting up from the hall didn't help: 'For you are always, close to me': 'I watch the sunrise'.

I was asked by a mum today if the rumour was true that I was retiring at Christmas! She said, 'Thank God you're not – you're too young to sit at home and vegetate.' How old do they think I am?

Saturday 9th

I pick up my pen and am not really sure what to write. Jo and Matt have chosen an engagement ring today. It should be ready next Friday. Six months to the day tomorrow – Tuesday will be the date – Shaun died. Six months which I suppose have gone quickly. People have helped tremendously. Six months without my man – I still feel so raw. Saw Steve and Mary. She is obviously more with it than she was in the week. Spoke to Kath later on, she says the boys have been told that their mother is dying – but she couldn't talk as obviously Mary was within earshot.

The turf has been laid on Kathleen's grave – the topsoil has been put on Shaun's. Comforting for Kathleen – almost as though she has an extra blanket for the cold weather.

A quote from Raymond Baxter during the Festival of Remembrance: 'Time is remorseless. Time inevitably brings change. But remembrance lives on.' How true.

Six Months

Sunday 10th

Six months to the day without my man. Six months sounds a long time – in fact it has gone quickly. Obviously because life has been so busy. I think I have become a good actress – playing a part on the surface, but God, I miss him so much. Why did it have to be us? We jogged along together through life. Knowing each other inside out really. Now it has gone, that companionship and loyalty.

How have I gone through the last six months? God has played a big, big part. I don't care to think how I would have been without faith, without having the certain knowledge that there is a Heaven and that Shaun is there. I think I would have just given up.

Matt played his first game of rugby today, for Medway fifths. Read at Mass tonight. Remembrance Sunday.

Monday 11th

10.30 p.m.: I have just asked Shaun to make Mary's passing easy, beautiful and peaceful. He did it for us: I would like Shaun to do it for Steve and the boys. Steve phoned earlier. Mary had been alright during the day but this evening Nick, her eldest son, was in talking to her and Steve said he appeared, white-faced, saying she was talking gibberish. Steve said she was getting frustrated because she couldn't make herself understood. It was worse when she tried to write – she kept repeating the words 'up, up, up' as she wrote. Nick was upset – didn't want to go to school. Steve has told him to speak to me if he is upset. Will Mary join Shaun tomorrow – six months – or will she be alright again in the morning? God is the only one who knows.

Tuesday 12th

School Mass was for Shaun. Appropriate by the date. Spoke to Steve, saw Breda at Mass at St Peter's and Fr Chris went to give Mary communion. She has had what would have appeared in other circumstances to be a stroke. Apparently it is the tumour attacking the part of the brain which deals with speech.

A couple of things said at the bereavement meeting: the guilt feeling after you have been happy for a little while, and how you miss the hugs.

Friday 15th

What to write? I haven't written for a few days because I only have the same things to say; loneliness really – utter loneliness.

Jo has her engagement ring today – it is beautiful. They have gone out for a meal tonight. I look at them and it transports me back. Funny, years go by yet in your head you do not really grow old. I hope they have longer together than we did. How can I climb out of this abyss? Shaun made me what I am and he is no longer here to help me carry on. I can't really get my true feelings down on paper. How can you explain how much you miss when your man has gone?

Saturday 16th

Quote from a letter in *The Universe* newspaper:

'The trouble about life just now is that I seem to *have* all the things that don't matter and to have *lost* all the things that do matter. I have life, I have enough money to live on, I have plenty to occupy me, but I am alone and sometimes I feel that nothing can make up for that.'

Sunday 17th

Hank and Anne have been today. Steve, Jo's brother, joined us for dinner.

A nice day, but it is hard to have a nice day with Shaun missing. He used to enjoy these get-togethers.

I thought people said the loss would lessen? It hasn't. I couldn't really care less whether I go on or not. Okay, looking after the boys, running the house and working all take time – and I think I am doing these alright – but at the end of the day it is the loneliness that gets you. That is what I could willingly do without.

Monday 18th

Nanna would have been 91 today. Staff Development Day in the museum which went very well.

Parish proposals for new church consultation meeting tonight. Didn't finish until nearly 10.00 p.m. I think it was almost in favour of a new building.

Could it be my fault that Shaun had to die? I think it has made me a more caring person – is that the reason why? 'Then shall I know.'

Tuesday 19th

New arrivals at school today. Irish travellers. I got upset when I arrived home tonight. The pyracantha had come away from the wall and was hanging over the front of the door. I have tried to tie it back. I know it took Shaun hours to do it. I am not so strong or tall as he was. I think I can cope without him and then something like this comes along and I know I can't do everything.

Spoke to Steve – things the same. However, Mary is on only 2–3 millilitres of liquid morphine as opposed to Shaun's 16 mls.

I feel down, tired, miserable; the bad weather doesn't help. I feel alone without my partner. I'm waking up once or twice a night now. Not a real problem – I go back to sleep – but having disturbed nights must make me more tired. Yet, I can't go to bed early; I'm afraid of staying awake. I **know** what I need, and I can't have it.

11.45 p.m.: What does God expect widows to do? What does he hope they would do? What are his plans for them? I would love to scan the Bible, Old and New Testaments, to try and find out. Monogamy must come into it.

Wednesday 20th

Jo and I went to see the Bridgewood Hotel tonight with regard to the wedding. Very impressed – but it is going to cost. What a shame Shaun will never see the wedding, will never see his sons get married. Life is still so unreal – I still expect to see him again. I need him to calm me down and put me in my place. I want my man. There is one sure thing about life: it isn't fair! It deals blows you really don't expect.

Apart from missing Shaun as a person and for all the personal reasons – I miss having someone to share the responsibility with.

I have to make all the decisions without a second opinion, someone to discuss things with – someone to tell me if I'm on the wrong track. Miss him, miss him, miss him.

Thursday 21st

I look at Shaun's photo and then have this vision of him decaying in his coffin. It is not right. I know it is only his body – but I loved his body as well. It is not fair. *I* need him. Why did God want him yet?

Have had Open Night at school tonight so I suppose I'm tired. I was fine but I shed a few tears later talking to a friend – one of the parents, Tess L. G.

Sunday 24th

Mary died early this morning. I feel so helpless – I can only talk and offer practical advice. Steve is devastated – half of his married life has been dogged by Mary's cancer.

What a weekend. I had been over there yesterday and the doctor had been to give her an injection to try to clear the pain. She was asleep while I was there. Steve was very tired.

Had a lovely evening at The Hengist last night with Terry, Geraldine and Fr Jim. Didn't go to bed until nearly 2.00 a.m.

Up early for the special *Christ the King* Feast Day Mass. It was so well done. The children took up a paper rose to be pinned on a tree with the names of all the people of the parish who had died this year. Very moving and tears were shed. Then to get the news of Mary – I have been over twice. Went to see Breda afterwards.

Monday 25th

Heavy feeling sort of day. Janet was upset at school and then apologised for me having to comfort her! Maybe this is my role. I really do not mind.

Went to Steve's. Read to the boys while Steve and his mother and brother (Kath and Paul) had their dinner. Was there longer than I thought. Steve has been to the undertakers and the Registrar – found it hard. He is having Mary buried in her wedding dress and long, large earrings. A nice idea. He had a few tears – he will shed many more – but it was a nice evening. Mary is to be buried in Holy Cross Churchyard at Bearsted. Steve goes running past there so he will be able to stop and say 'hello'. A nice memory for him.

Wednesday 27th

Midnight: What is there to say? I have been home for an hour – had a very nice evening in Raffles with Paul and Brenda. Shaun is very much missed.

David Cunningham was on the news tonight. The Hickman line pump is beginning to save lives. I knew Shaun was here on earth for a purpose! I know it is sad that it wasn't someone else's purpose to go through the treatment to save him. He went through it to help others. His comment of September 24th last year – 'if anything experimental is offered, I will take it, either for me or for others' – has come true!

Spoke to Steve. He is getting unwarranted hassle from the DHSS. Saw him after school yesterday with Mary's Mum and sister. **What** is he going through? I do know. He is going to see Mary tomorrow in the Chapel of Rest.

All of a sudden I am crying – why is my man not here to help me? Why? If the treatment had been developed a year earlier would it have made a difference? I know it is right that things are learned through different treatments – and that things are modified – but if this had happened to us two years into the future, would maybe things have been alright? I really do hope so for the patients who will be at that stage then, but it is hard to think that, physically, you could have been so near the breakthrough – that for what is just a matter of months, really, Shaun has missed out. Not just Shaun – all of us.

Thursday 28th

The first of Mary's funeral Masses tonight. Steve stood up well with the boys, but he was pale and drawn. Kath broke down afterwards. During the last hymn – 'I watch the sunrise' – I could almost *feel* that Shaun had his arms round Mary.

Sue had contacted the DHSS for me. Steve is not entitled to the £1000 or a widower's pension. Surely this is discrimination?

Friday 29th

11.30 p.m.: Have put off writing this page until late. Probably the most raw day for six months. The church was packed. Saw Des and Sini – friends through rugby – beforehand. The Lourdes hymn was sung –

and 'I watch the sunrise' – but Mary's sister also read out the Weaver's Prayer. Probably this was the day when I couldn't keep my outside face on – it was too much! Yet during the Weaver's Prayer I could feel Shaun smiling at us all with his arms around Mary – even though I wanted his arms around me. I broke down almost completely at the end. Thought I'd pulled myself together outside until I felt someone put his arms around me. John H. I had forgotten he knew Steve and would be there – he was surprised to see me. I'm afraid I just sobbed into his shirt. I did ring to apologise tonight. Went back into school, still crying. Mr D. was good – knew it was better for me to get back to the kids. The teacher for the traveller children was in class. Anyway, the kids were pretty good. After 10 minutes the Portuguese lad asked why my eyes were red. I just said, 'Tears'. He was puzzled until someone said, 'Of course they're tears. She's been to a funeral.' The traveller girl mouthed across the room to me: 'Are you alright?' She later looked at my locket and said, 'That is your man – no wonder you are upset.' An eight-year-old with deep perception.

What do I say to Steve tomorrow? Is it right to go? It is *for me* – but is it *for them*?

I went back to 12.30 p.m. Mass, as it was for Shaun. I sat two rows in front of where I'd sat earlier – and on the bench was a blue balloon. What can I read into that? I left it. Not green, but blue – for Mary? I wish now I had taken it.

Saturday 30th

10.55 p.m.: Went to the cemetery. They have laid the turf. Shaun has his overcoat on for the winter! Went to Holy Cross afterwards to see Mary's.

Fr Jim said tonight that he went to the cemetery today but went in the other entrance – didn't see my car, so left! A pity. Went over to Steve's. His father (Buck), Kath, Paul and sister-in-law Fiona were there. They are okay. Relieved I think that things are over.

I asked Steve who chose the Weaver's Prayer. He smiled and said he *thought* I'd like it.

Apparently Micky Skinner, the England rugby player, had been good with the boys yesterday. He signed autographs and played pillow fights. He is talking about getting a signed (England) rugby ball for Steve to raffle for the Marsden.

16

Life Goes On

Monday 2nd

7.30 p.m.: Should we keep the words 'for ever'? How can anything be promised for ever? How can anything last for ever – except God – and love?? – and hurt??

Have been out with Rose and Catherine tonight. Muswells – a nice evening.

Went to Mum's yesterday. Saw Florrie first, then Nick and Sue and Dave and Mary arrived at Mum's. Nice.

Wednesday 4th

Steve brought my wine tonight. Arrived fairly early. I wasn't composed enough for him. He is hurting – my God, I know how much. Talking to him about whether I should still see him and his family. He said he didn't think he could have done what I had over the last few months. **But** what they don't understand is that I am selfish and am taking from them – not **giving**. I feel they do me good. I can relate to them. Why has this happened to us? World concern over Aids. But 90% is self-inflicted. Not like cancer.

Sunday 8th

Haven't written for a few days. Been fairly down. Out with Alice on
Thursday to The Wheelers. On Friday Fr Jim phoned and got me
through a bad patch before I went to the convent for a social with the
Hythe group. Ian and Linda brought their video camera down on
Saturday so that we could borrow it for the Australia trip, and we
went to the Running Horse for a meal.

This morning Jo and I went to the Tudor Park – think this is where
they will have their wedding reception. They then took the car as Matt
was playing rugby. Stuart and I walked to town. Met Fr Jim and he
later phoned. He is really good – he took me out for a drink to the
Imperial at Hythe. We walked along the front. Very bracing, a lovely
evening – lots of conversation. Funny, I've seen the sea only twice
this year – apart from flying over it to and from Lourdes – and both
times have been at night with Fr Jim among others.

Had a peculiar dream last night. I was driving the new car – just
Shaun and me – through a wood on a narrow road, and suddenly I
had to stop because the wood gave way to what was a cliff. If I
had gone further the car would probably have upended. I certainly
wouldn't have got it back up. It was a beach cove in Cornwall –
nowhere I think Shaun and I had ever been. Funny, I want so much
to dream of him – although this one was rather disappointing. We
just chatted on the drive, about nothing in particular, I think, because
I cannot remember it.

Monday 9th

IT/DT* Staff Development Day today plus parent/governor meeting
tonight. Five parents only. We all went into the presbytery afterwards
with Fr Jim for coffee. Got home to a phone call from Julie C. – John's
mother died this morning. The funeral is on Monday so I don't think I
will be able to get there.

Elizabeth phoned. Lionel is not well – won't be driving us to Heathrow. Heathrow? Shaun drove me there two years ago so I could go to
Canada on a teacher-exchange fortnight. Bittersweet. That couldn't
have caused his cancer could it? Me going away? He wanted me to

* Information Technology/Design Technology.

go, although with hindsight I don't think he was happy while I was away.

Spoke to Steve. Yesterday Micky Skinner came up trumps for him and the boys. Today, he is on his own – slept in his own bed for the first time in months. Loneliness, unreality – I identify with him. A swear word here. That is what earthly life is. Shaun, help me.

Wednesday 11th

Fr Chris and the bereavement meeting last night. Special Mass for Mary's friends.

Steve has had a few days of physical work which will do him good – gets him through being on his own.

Actually had an evening in. Wrapped presents, stripped the bed after the hot-water-bottle burst last night. Many phone calls, including Roger, who will take us to Heathrow. He did so much driving for Shaun and now he will do it for us. I don't know what I feel. Perverse really – I know I don't want to be here. I don't want 'our' Christmas. But I don't want to leave the grave unattended either. I go without any feelings.

Spoke to David, Rose's husband, tonight. Something he said, a saying of his mother's – 'While you are marching you can't fight.' In other words, keep busy. I do that as much as I can, but even now (one day off seven months) it is sometimes unreal – Shaun will still come back.

Friday 13th

5.15 p.m.: Last day at school. It has suddenly hit me that I am going away. I have now changed from not caring at all two days ago to being positively anti-going. I'm frightened really – losing my security because Shaun is *here*. Well, I can't back out. Steve delivered wine last night – late. He had been to help a friend of Mary's who had had an accident. He has been working for a few days. Better for him. They were burgled on Sunday evening – while he and the boys were there. Steve had £40 taken with his wallet and Kath's handbag had £200 Christmas money in it. What else can go wrong for them?

Going to St Simon Stock's Carol Concert later.

Saturday 14th

Had 6.00 p.m. Mass said as a Christmas present for Shaun. Beautiful morning today. So clear and cold. The trees! All the branches absolutely hanging with frost. So cold at the cemetery. The water had frozen and I had a job to replace the flowers. Spoke to Shaun – told him I would see him in three weeks at the most. Could be sooner of course if anything happens. Wouldn't wish that on anyone else except myself, though.

Josephine has been. Was talking to her about priorities and you tend to put pleasure at the bottom. I learned *that* last September – Shaun came first then. Before it was work and chores to be done before you could allow yourself the pleasurable bits.

Shock in Mass tonight. Peter H. died in the early hours of the morning. Spoke to Sr Mary – before now, I don't think any of the people who had been on the Lourdes trips with this group had died.

Sunday 15th

Nick and Sue brought Mum and Dad down this morning. They visited the cemetery first. Sue and Mum more upset when they went. Kelly called in. Fr Jim called in tonight to wish us 'Bon Voyage'.

We had a sort of Christmas dinner with presents tonight. Steve phoned – had to promise him no postcard!

I hope I'm doing the right thing going away – I'm frightened really of losing the security of *here* where Shaun is. He will come with me I hope. Not Christmas – summer holiday. I think when I get back I will be able to say, 'Well, I did it and enjoyed it.' I have to move forward. My life has got to change – mustn't live in the past. I let Shaun go, I must go on. I know he wouldn't have wanted this suffering and loneliness for us.

Postscript

January 1992

Well, I did do it! And I did enjoy it! But I was glad to get back having done it. Does that make sense? The journey out to Singapore, with the lights of Istanbul from 10,000 feet and sunrise over the Caucasus mountains at 3.15 a.m. (according to my body clock) was breathtaking. Singapore – with its authentic Chinese meals, balmy temperatures and wealth of shops – I very much enjoyed, even though the boys weren't into shopping. Something I probably won't experience again. Sitting in a hotel bedroom on my own was a first. Funny how all hotel bedrooms have identical room layouts. You could be almost anywhere – they look the same. It could have been Stratford or Oxford or Paris – all the hotel weekend breaks I shared with Shaun over the years. With Singapore, I was on my own. Still, I did it. I could almost hear Shaun saying, 'Go for it, girl.'

We were thoroughly spoiled by Mike and Jill in Perth. What would Shaun have made of it all? It wasn't a bit like Christmas. Blue skies, summer clothes, high temperatures. I couldn't, wouldn't, didn't want to get into the Christmas feeling. This was to be a summer holiday. Not exactly the one Shaun and I had planned for Northern Ireland. I hope he approved of me being here. I felt really relaxed while away – a combination of being well looked after and sunny skies, and spent a lot of time just reading. Actually, without realising it, I had chosen my novels rather well. I want to add a couple more quotes here which I found particularly relevant. They are all from *September* by Rosamunde Pilcher.

'Grief is a funny thing, because you don't have to carry it with you for the rest of your life. After a bit you set it down by the roadside and walk on and leave it resting there.'

Will this really happen? Will I be able one day to set down my grief without guilt and just keep within me the happy memories? It would be nice.

'And one day, sooner or later, you'll meet someone. Someone just as special as you are. She won't fill Mary's place, because she'll have a place of her own. And she'll fill it for all the right reasons.'

That quote might help Steve.

'Never lose sight of the fact that, beyond the winter, a new spring was already on its way.'

I think the essence of that last quote was what lay behind my writing this diary. I know, and have said, that I need to go forward. Things will gradually improve – they will have to. Positive thinking. But no one can help with that. It is something which I will have to work out for myself. It won't happen overnight, I know that. I must still expect the down moments; it is still such early days, but, if I can make myself hang on to the thought of a spring around the corner, then, even if it is not meant to be this chronological spring, one will come for me – even if it is out of season. Rather like a bonus.

A Lesson to be Learned

If I had my time again, I would throw away the rules. I lived by the rule book. You have children, and your duty is to them. Later you can get back to what you originally had with your husband – only (and I looked forward to that time with longing) we never made it. I would advise anyone **not** to do it the way I did, even if at the time it seems so right – because you never know what God has in store for you. I suppose what I am saying is: 'live for the present. Make the most of what you have got.'

Actually, it is easy to say I would throw away the rule book. I know deep down that I couldn't really do that. I don't regret a minute of the life we shared. The boys were a bonus to us. They made us what we became. And it was good. Shaun lives on through them.

Now it is up to me. I don't want people to do things for me. I've always coped, and I don't want that taken away from me – the thought of someone else running my life makes me edgy. People want to take care of those who are hurt – but I want to cope. It is now down to me.

Reference

Rosamunde Pilcher (1991) *September*, Coronet Books; reproduced by permission of Hodder & Stoughton Ltd., London.